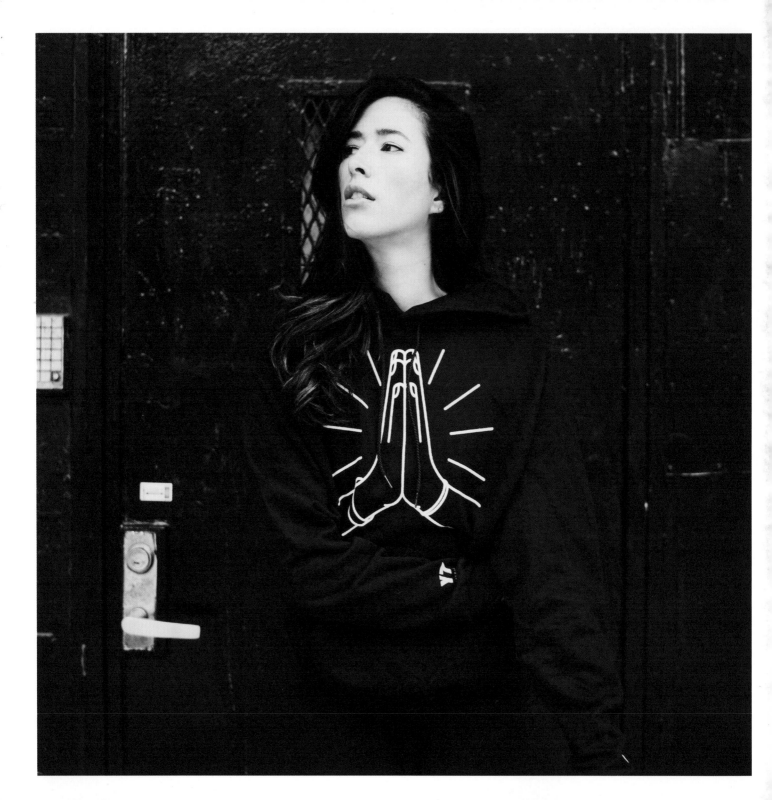

WE FLOW HARD

The Y7 Guide to Crafting
Your Yoga Practice

by **Sarah and Mason Levey**
cofounders of Y7 Studio

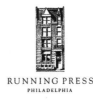

RUNNING PRESS
PHILADELPHIA

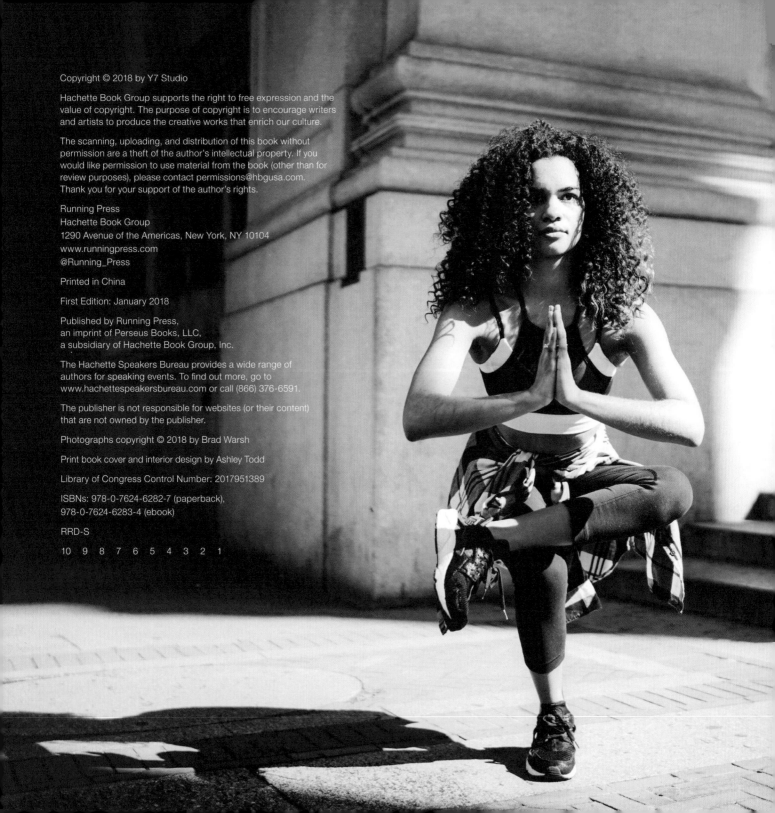

Running Press
Hachette Book Group
1290 Avenue of the Americas, New York, NY 10104
www.runningpress.com
@Running_Press

Printed in China

First Edition: January 2018

Published by Running Press,
an imprint of Perseus Books, LLC,
a subsidiary of Hachette Book Group, Inc.

The Hachette Speakers Bureau provides a wide range of authors for speaking events. To find out more, go to www.hachettespeakersbureau.com or call (866) 376-6591.

The publisher is not responsible for websites (or their content) that are not owned by the publisher.

Photographs copyright © 2018 by Brad Warsh

Print book cover and interior design by Ashley Todd

Library of Congress Control Number: 2017951389

ISBNs: 978-0-7624-6282-7 (paperback),
978-0-7624-6283-4 (ebook)

RRD-S

10 9 8 7 6 5 4 3 2 1

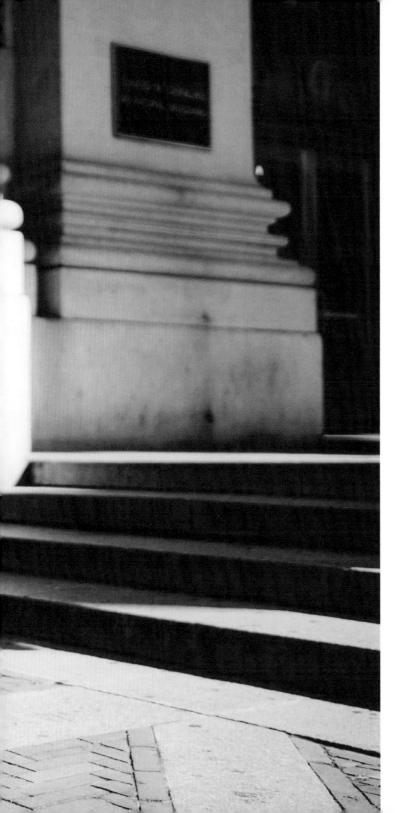

Contents

Foreword 6

Part 1: Foundation 8
    THE BEGINNING 10
    THE PHILOSOPHY 16
    THE PAYOFF 20

Part 2: Flow 28
    SWEAT-DRIPPING, BEAT-BUMPING, CANDLELIT YOGA 30
    FINDING YOUR BEATS 38
    STRIKE A POSE 54
    WARM-UP SEQUENCE 58
    Y7 FLOW 76
    Y7 MEGA DETOX 96
    ABS & ASS SEQUENCE 112

Part 3: Namast'ay Fly 128
    FINDING BALANCE 130
    CARING FOR YOUR BODY 150
    NOURISHING YOUR MIND 168

Afterword 192
Acknowledgments 195
Pose Glossary 196
Index 201

FOREWORD

I started going to Y7 a few years ago—

after I modeled for the *Sports Illustrated Swimsuit Edition* and received a month-long free pass to the studio inside of their gift bag. Even though I began practicing yoga in the Hudson Valley, where I grew up, I had yet to find a studio in New York that made me feel at home—so I decided to give Y7 a try. During my first class I knew right away that Y7 was the place for me. For the first time in a long time my yoga practice felt like my own. The energy was both high and grounding at the same time, which was a balance I had always craved from my practice. After my first class, I started going every day. Y7 felt like a gift I was giving myself and I couldn't get enough of it.

My favorite thing about Y7 is that after every single class I take, I walk away feeling balanced, centered, and energized. From my perspective, Y7 is unique because every single teacher and student is on the same page about what the community wants. Each teacher leads the class through a high energy, supportive practice—and class is centered on checking in with yourself, grounding yourself, and moving in a way that feels good for you. Y7 encourages you to figure out what you need each day, and the dark, candlelit room allows you to move in a way that is completely your own. The mirrorless rooms also allowed me to really check in with myself—at Y7 I stopped focusing on how I was looking, or if I was in the correct pose, and instead began to finally get in touch with what was going on inside.

The community at Y7 is one of inclusivity and celebration. What I love about Y7 is that there is no air of what practicing yoga *should be* or *look like*. Instead, the community celebrates and encourages all of the different groups of people who simply want to practice yoga, have fun, and do something good for themselves. For a while, there has been a certain idea of what a yogi or yoga in general is supposed to be and I think Y7 has completely changed that. In creating a book about the Y7 experience, Sarah and Mason are creating a way for people who might not have access to a studio to feel included in the Y7 community and encouraged to deepen their practice in a way that feels good to them.

—Emily DiDonato

PART 1

Foun-
dation

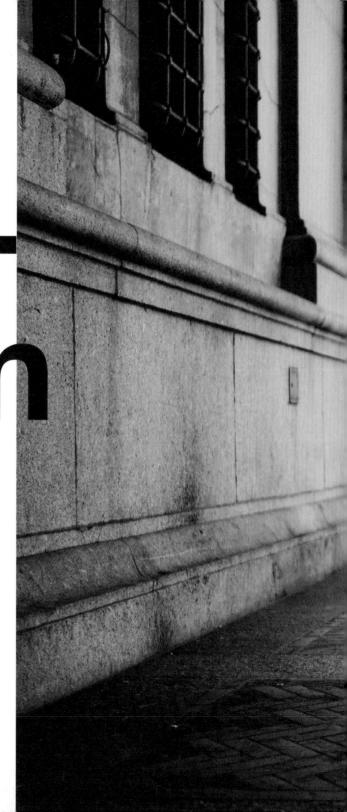

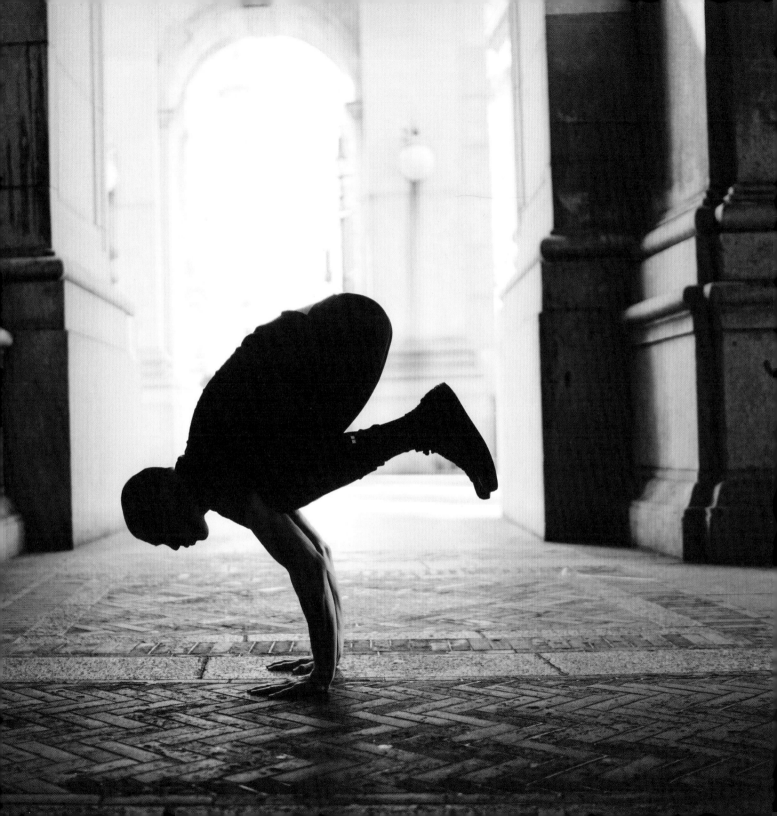

THE
BEGINNING

To really understand Y7, it helps to know how we started and where we came from. We didn't set out to start a yoga studio. Not really, anyway. The process was more organic than that, growing out of our own experiences and frustrations with practicing in more traditional environments. We've always been creative people, and building Y7 ourselves was the natural answer to the question we seemed to always come back to: how could we practice yoga in a way that felt exciting and authentic, with good energy, good music, and good people?

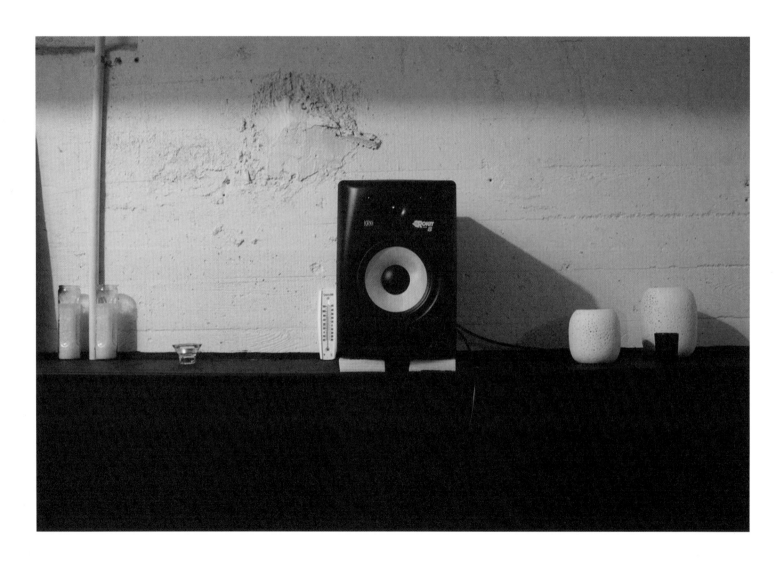

I had practiced on and off for about five years, but no matter which classes I took, I always left feeling like something was missing—that I needed to go to the gym or take another cardio-based class to get a complete workout. I wasn't getting the physical payoff I wanted for my body, and I wasn't getting the studio experience I wanted in my life. To be honest, I really felt like I was wasting time and money, and as a result, for a while I stopped practicing altogether.

My husband was always a more consistent yogi than I was, but he wasn't satisfied with traditional studios either. We couldn't find a place that combined the passion we had for yoga with the intense workout we were looking for. And we definitely couldn't find a place to practice that had the right vibe, that felt like *us*. After dealing with the same frustrations over and over again, we decided to do something about it—and that's when we created the concept of Y7.

We actually started Y7 as a pop-up in July 2013. Before we had studios or staff, it was just me and Mason setting up shop in a huge room in Williamsburg, Brooklyn. We rented the space for a few hours one weekend from a recording studio that wasn't using it. All of our classes were free.

You should have seen us: me and my now-husband trekking down Bedford Avenue to the temporary studio with two *huge* rolling trunks full of supplies. And then, in the middle of the summer heat, lugging those trunks up to the fourth-floor walk-up. The first weekend we had no idea who would show up, what the reception would be, or if people would even like what we were doing. It was a complete unknown, but it was also incredibly exciting.

At the end of that weekend, someone asked us for a studio schedule and wanted to know if they could buy a package of classes. And that was all it took. That one person showing interest and loving what we had created was enough for us to say, *okay, maybe we can do this*.

We continued Y7 as a pop-up until September 2013, when we found a 300-square-foot space in Williamsburg we could afford on our salaries. At that time, we both still had full-time jobs—I was an account executive working in fashion, and Mason was working in digital advertising. We couldn't believe there were people who wanted to practice yoga the way we did and who wanted to spend their free time practicing with us in the space we were so proud of. Looking back, that was the beginning of our tribe of yogis.

It wasn't all perfect. There were days when that conviction in our mission and our tribe faltered. Some days, not a single person would show up to the 7:00 p.m. class, and we would close early. Fall/Winter 2013 was rough for us, balancing our jobs, our lives, and our fledgling studio. Most of my days looked like this:

5:45 A.M.	**WAKE UP (ACCOUNT FOR SNOOZE BUTTON TIME)**
6:15 A.M.	**ARRIVE AT THE STUDIO TO GET THE ROOM READY, CHECK PEOPLE IN, ETC.**
7:00–8:00 A.M.	**EITHER TAKE CLASS OR HANG OUT UNTIL CLASS WAS OVER**
8:15 A.M.	**HAND THE STUDIO KEYS OVER TO MY INSTRUCTOR, SO I COULD GO TO WORK**
9:00 A.M.–6:00 P.M.	**DAY-JOB GRIND**
6:00 P.M.	**LEAVE THE OFFICE AS FAST AS I COULD IN ORDER TO GET BACK TO THE STUDIO TO SET UP AND CHECK PEOPLE IN FOR EVENING CLASSES**
9:30 P.M.	**CLOSE UP AND GO HOME**

It was brutal and certainly didn't leave a lot of room for anything else. Sometimes Mason and I would switch off responsibilities or take turns monitoring the different classes, but this schedule is just a little glimpse of what our lives were like until the spring of 2015. During that year and a half of building Y7 and working full-time, we hustled hard and planned for the company's future. As we saw our class slots filling up and our waitlists

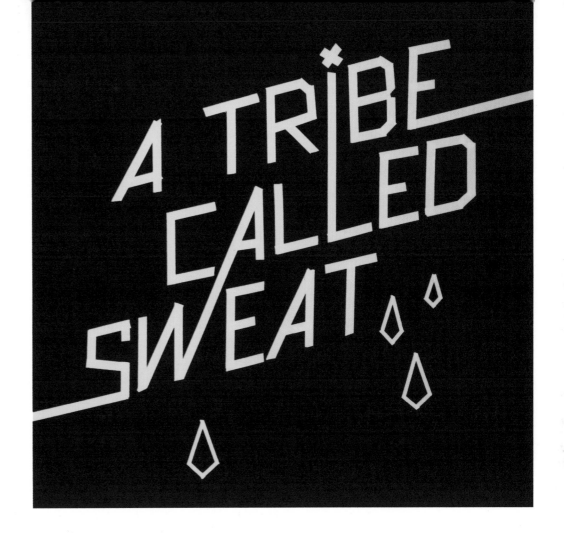

growing, we knew we had to expand. It took a lot of savings (I actually called my parents and had them cash in my savings bonds), time, and sleepless nights to figure out how to get into Manhattan. Finally, in January 2015 we popped up in SoHo for seven months.

In the spring of 2015, we opened the Flatiron district location of Y7—our third studio. At that point, we were so proud of what we had built, and we were finally able to quit our jobs and dedicate everything we have to Y7, creating spaces for our tribe to learn and grow.

THE
PHILOSOPHY

WHAT WE DO (AND WHY WE DO IT)

When we were first thinking about Y7, I drew inspiration from those whose practices I admired. The yoga teacher Rachel Brathen really impacted me when she said, "The yoga pose is not the goal. Becoming flexible or standing on your hands is not the goal. The goal is to create space where you were once stuck. To unveil layers of protection you've built around your heart. To appreciate your body and become aware of the mind and the noise it can create. To make peace with who you are."

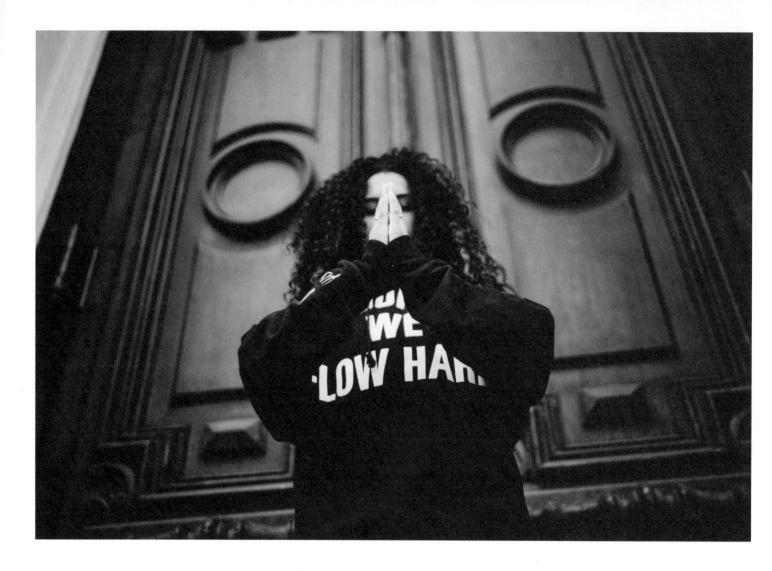

We knew we didn't want our studio to be like every other studio out there. We wanted a practice with music we wanted to listen to, music that inspired us. We wanted to sweat and move. We wanted a place where people could practice and not be worried about what the person next to them looked like, to fall and not care. Most of all, we wanted a place to be ourselves and get deeper into our own individual practices. We saw a void in the market and decided to fill it.

The bottom line is: people are busy. We wanted to provide a yoga experience that would make people sweat, really using their muscles and giving them a good workout. The physical component of our studio was always at the forefront of our minds. But we also wanted to maintain the basic teachings and spiritual aspect of the practice. In blending these two fundamental ideals, we have built up an amazing tribe of yogis who support and challenge each other.

To achieve these goals, we decided to set up our studios in a very specific way. The design and feel of the studios are all black and white, with minimal furniture and plants—we wanted everything really clean and simple. We decided to take out the mirrors you'd typically find in a yoga studio, and we made the space intentionally dark, illuminated with just candlelight, so that our clients can feel comfortable to move in their own way and not worry about whether anyone else can see them. We also heat the rooms, to really get the sweat going and the body moving.

During yoga sessions, the music and the beat drive the breath that cues the poses. This environmental setup leads into the way we've structured our classes. We practice one breath to one movement, building up heat within the body. In our classes, instructors teach the sequences and then allow the students to flow through them on their own. We believe that you should be able to make the flow yours—if something doesn't feel good on your body, take it out. You want to try that handstand hop a couple more times? Do it. Your yoga practice is your own, and you should feel encouraged to modify what you are doing to make it that way.

We believe in being yourself, in embracing your body and not forcing yourself into the preconceived notions of a shape, pose, or lifestyle. What works for you may not work for someone else. At our studios, and with this book, we want you to come as you are with all of your flaws, feelings, or not . . . it is up to you. All we want is for you to be open and the rest will come.

THE
PAYOFF

Our tribe of yogis is made up of people who practice yoga for a lot of different reasons. One of the things we love best about our practice is that it attracts people with unique goals for their mental, physical, and spiritual well-being. Whether you're someone who has been practicing yoga for years, someone who has tried it out a few times and wasn't sure, or someone who has never hit the mat before, we welcome you.

There are as many reasons why yogis choose to start a yoga practice as there are yogis. Some reasons come up over and over again, though, whether we're at the studio, conducting a workshop, or talking to people we meet in our day-to-day lives. You've probably considered some of these reasons yourself. Maybe your goal is weight loss, or increasing flexibility, or promoting general health, or working your way toward enlightenment . . . well, *maybe*. Whatever reasons you may have for beginning your practice, they are your own.

Regardless of your specific motivations, there are several benefits that will usually come from practicing yoga, whether you plan for them or not:

1 **STRESS RELIEF:** By starting a yoga practice, you are taking time for yourself and recognizing your body in a way that is both mindful and joyful. It is a great way to get rid of the stress that can accumulate daily in both the mind and the body—because even when we believe we have stress under control mentally, our bodies often hold on to it. During your practice, whether by yourself or in a group, you are encouraged to clear your mind, focus on the breath, and get out of that stressful sitting position that you may be in all day at your desk.

2 **WEIGHT LOSS:** Fast-paced and heated practices, such as vinyasa and Bikram, are examples of the types of yoga that can be beneficial for weight loss. However, if you incorporate a regular practice—of any sort—into your life, your body will become stronger and more tuned to what it needs. That kind of focused attention on the body, combined with the natural strength training of a yoga practice, can also help eliminate cravings you may have had before.

3 **OVERALL HEALTH:** This may seem obvious, but it is also the most essential benefit of yoga: you are the happiest and healthiest when you are balanced in your mind and body. Health is not only about being physically fit, but also maintaining emotional and mental balance. Yoga gives us a

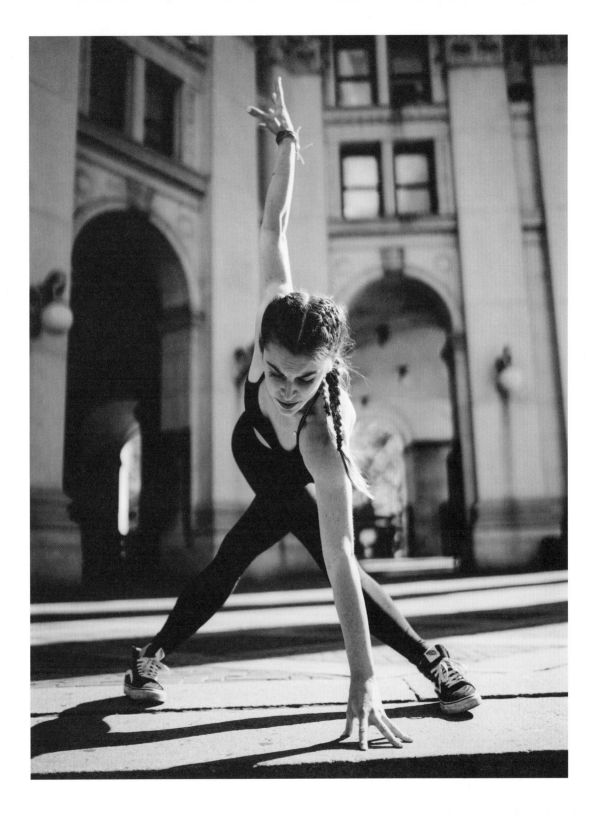

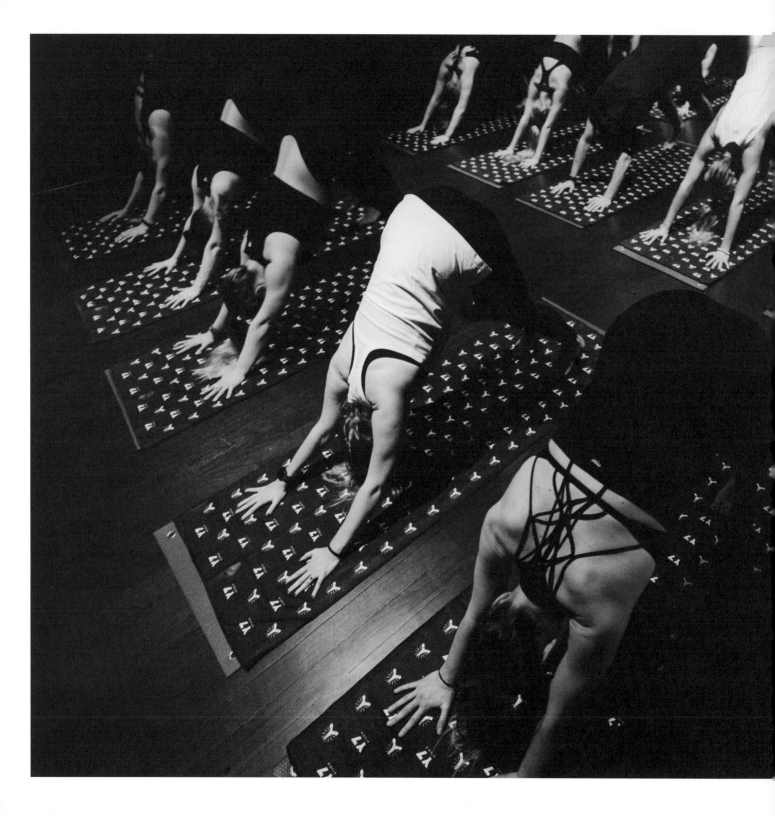

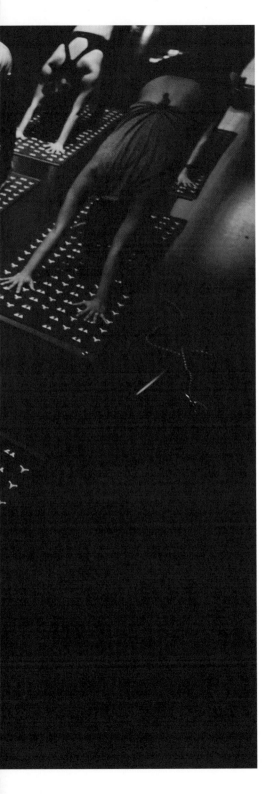

place not just to sweat, but to acknowledge the link between our mind and body, honoring that space and contributing to an overall sense of well-being.

4   GREATER AWARENESS: The mind is constantly involved in activity—swinging from the past to the future, but never taking time to stay in the present. By simply being aware of this tendency, we can actually save ourselves from getting stressed or worked up. Unplugging and being in the moment are the simplest and most essential way to relax the mind. Yoga and controlled breathing help create that *awareness* and bring the mind back to the present moment, where it can stay happy and focused. This is why we pay attention to the breath so much in a yoga practice, and why we at Y7 use a vinyasa flow that links movement to breath. It's also one of the reasons we keep our studios dark and eliminate mirrors—seeing your reflection, or how others are practicing, can distract you from being fully in the moment.

5   INCREASED ENERGY: We are all so busy with our jobs, personal lives, side hustles (we can relate!), workouts—the day-to-day is often overwhelming, especially when you've got a lot you want to accomplish. Shuffling multiple things throughout the day can be exhausting. Practicing yoga on a regular basis can help balance out your mind, giving you the space you need to tackle multiple things on your agenda. By focusing on just one thing for the length of your yoga session—whether that's an hour in a class or a short sequence in your living room—you clear the way for clearer thinking for the rest of your day.

6   BETTER FLEXIBILITY AND POSTURE: *Duh.* Yoga is all about alignment, and including yoga in your routine leads to a body that is strong and flexible. A regular practice not only stretches and tones the body's muscles, it also improves your posture when you stand, sit, and walk.

7 BONE HEALTH: Yoga focuses on using the body and tools you already have. It's a practice that asks you to bring nothing besides yourself—that's one of the things we love about it. As you begin your practice, you'll notice that the postures are load-bearing, which means that instead of lifting weights you will be using your own body weight. This aspect of yoga doesn't just tone your muscles—it also strengthens the bones and keeps them healthy. A consistent practice can even help to prevent osteoporosis.

8 IMPROVED HEALTH/IMMUNITY: Our bodies are made up of incredibly complex systems, and they're all interconnected. The immune system in particular is an amazing web affected not just by what we put in our bodies, but also how we treat them. Those connections are everywhere: an irregularity in the body affects the mind, and a restlessness in the mind can manifest as an illness in the body. The physical aspect of yoga strengthens the muscles; breathing techniques and meditation release stress and calm the mind. These different benefits work together to improve our overall health and bolster our immunity to illnesses. You'll also find that the yoga practice aids in detoxing the organs—when you are in twisting poses, you are essentially compressing the organs in your midsection, which stimulates blood flow and improves digestion. This in turn can help your kidneys and liver process more efficiently.

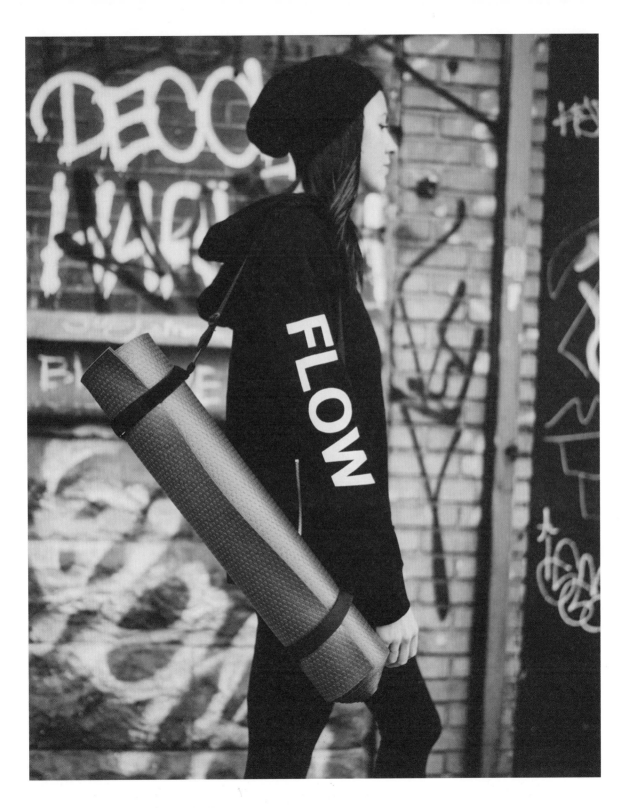

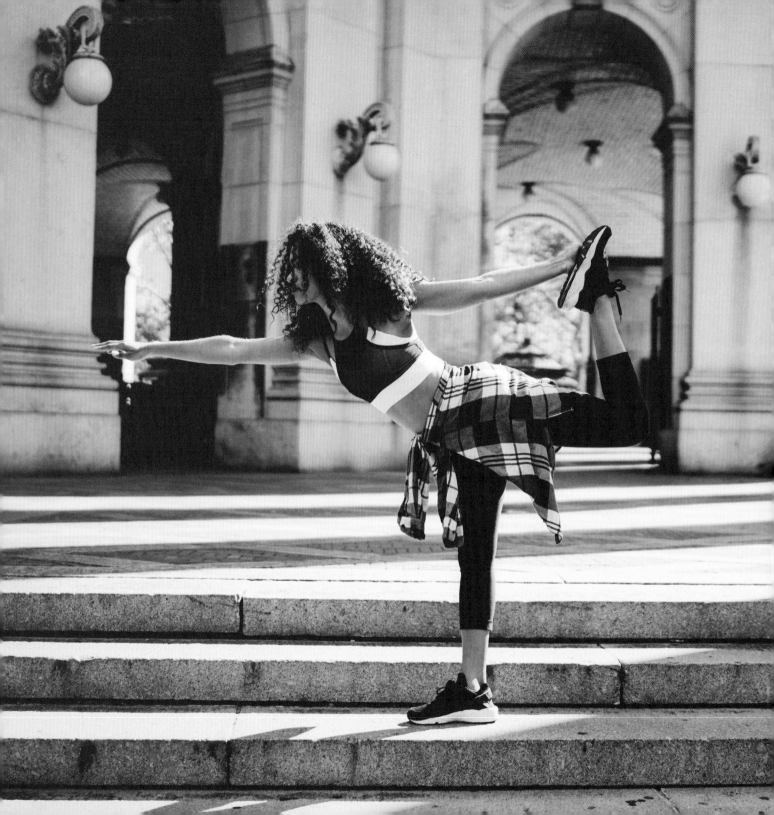

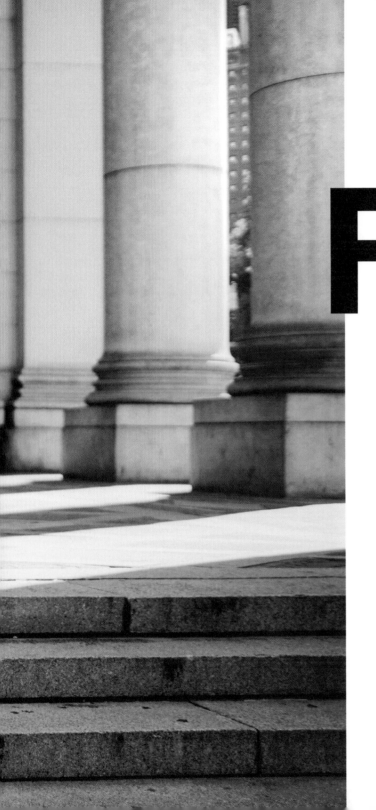

PART 2

Flow

SWEAT-DRIPPING BEAT-BUMPING CANDLELIT YOGA

Y7 is a very different approach to yoga, but it's rooted in the same traditions that have guided the practice for generations. To get a real sense of what makes hip-hop yoga distinct, it helps to have an understanding of the broader history of yoga.

Yoga is a 5,000-year-old practice that originated in India. The word itself is derived from the Sanskrit term *yuj*, which literally means "to bind." Today we interpret this as a way to unite—unite the body and the mind, unite the different areas of the body, unite with our fellow yogis. Although there are many schools of thought when it comes to practicing yoga (including Bikram, karma, ashtanga, vinyasa, kundalini, etc.), they all share the desire to harmonize the body and mind through breath and poses.

We often think about yoga as being one thing, but it is actually made up of eight interconnected limbs:

YAMAS (restraints)

NIYAMAS (observations)

ASANA (poses)

PRANAYAMA (breathing)

PRATYAHARA (withdrawal of senses)

DHARANA (concentration)

DHYANA (meditation)

SAMADHI (enlightenment)

When we practice yoga, we are encouraged to explore these eight limbs and begin refining our behavior, ultimately seeking to reach samadhi or enlightenment—*or* not. Not everyone has to have the goal of enlightenment when practicing yoga. At Y7, we don't expect our students and fellow yogis to come with a specific goal or agenda. We believe that just showing up on the mat is enough. Just opening yourself up to the ideas of yoga is enough. What you choose to do with what you discover is up to you.

Today most yogis are engaged in working on the third limb of yoga, asana, which is concerned with the progression of the physical postures. Even as just a physical practice, yoga is a unique experience. In our physical experience of yoga we work to connect the movement of the body and the fluctuations of the mind to the pattern of the breath. Connecting these distinct elements helps redirect our attention inward—instead of looking around at other practitioners' poses, or what they may look like, we concentrate entirely on our own practice in the moment. It is through this process of looking within that we learn to recognize our own habits and thought patterns without passing judgment on them. We become more aware of our experiences in the moment, and through cultivating that awareness we are able to progress more holistically, rather than fixating on the completion of a singular goal. It is this mind-body connection that we focus on at Y7.

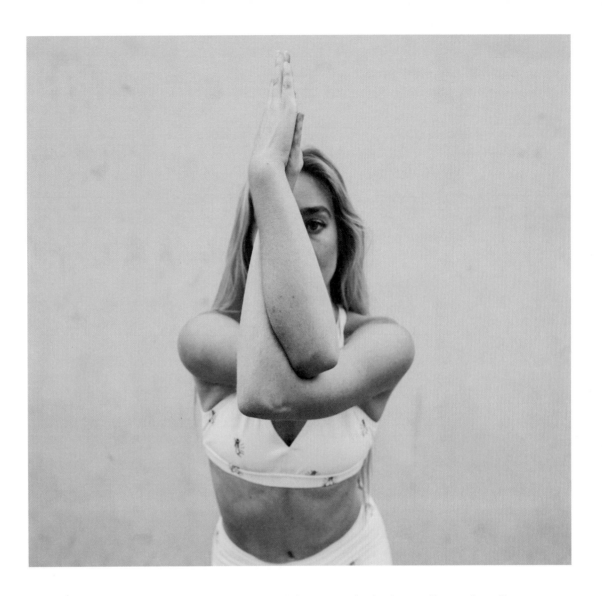

The vinyasa style of yoga—which we practice in the studios and you'll encounter in the sequences in this book—stems from the hatha practice. In a hatha practice students focus on finding the perfect alignment of the body in an asana. Vinyasa, which translates to "movement linked with breath," concentrates on the journey from pose to pose and the breath that connects those movements. Vinyasa practices today are

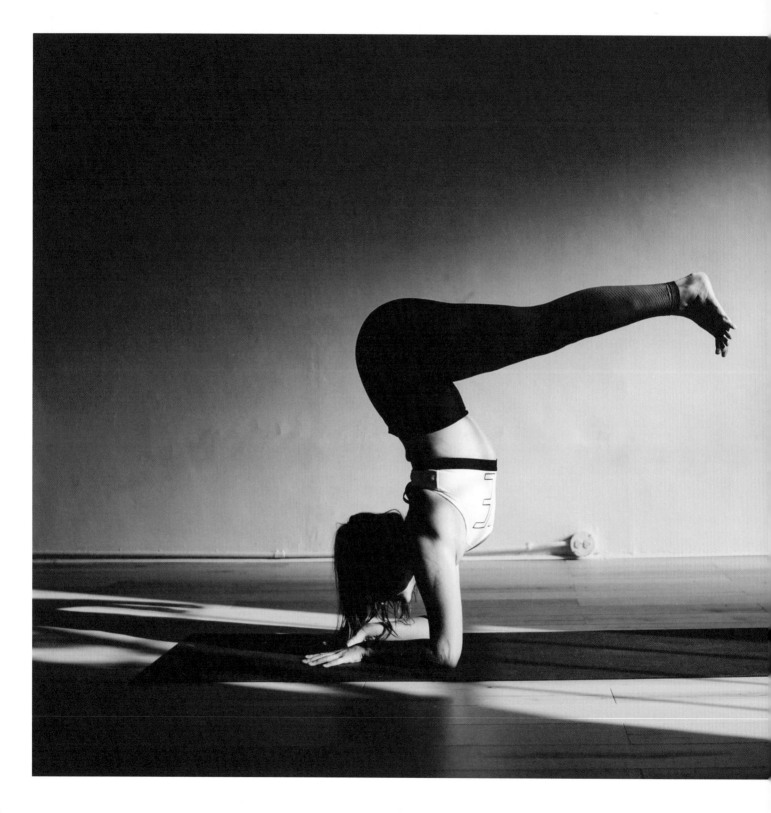

often quite dynamic; we like to refer to it as a moving meditation of sorts. The pace and the sequences can vary, as opposed to Bikram or ashtanga styles of yoga, which are more rigid in their routines. This dynamic aspect of vinyasa requires the mind to stay anchored in the present. At Y7 we guide our students through sequencing, cuing the breath, before allowing them to take that sequence and flow through it with their own individual breaths. This could mean taking the sequence at a slower pace with a more elongated breath; it could mean taking it faster; it could even mean eliminating a pose altogether if it is not serving you. The goal of this is to bring you closer to your body, zeroing in on the connection you have with yourself.

At Y7 we are dedicated to bringing the practice back to the individual—that's why we spend so much time creating an environment that is safe and inclusive. Everyone's body is different and everyone is at a different point in their journey—there is no reason to judge that. One of the most beautiful aspects of the practice is that the poses sustain and support you, no matter how fit you are at a given moment.

Ultimately, in our tribe when you come to the mat, you are there for yourself. When you enter the mirrorless, dark, candlelit room, we want you to forget all your preconceived notions about what yoga is supposed to be. When you enter this state, your body not only becomes stronger and more flexible—so does your mind.

WHY HIP-HOP?

As one of the founders of Y7, one of the questions I get asked the most is why hip-hop? Why include music in the practice, and why that particular type of music? The loud bass and the sometimes explicit lyrics make it seem like hip-hop would be the opposite of yoga. How do we make it work?

Cue the Y7 community.

When we set out to start our studios, right at the beginning it was clear that community would play a huge role in what we were doing. Over the years I have had the pleasure of getting to know a lot of our clients, and I've seen friendships form and bonds created—all brought together by this sweat-dripping, candlelit, beat-bumping yoga. And at the core of all of it are those beats . . . there is just something about them. When you hear hip-hop, you just want to move.

You can take the community of hip-hop way back to the block parties of the 1970s, when it was just groups of friends and families partying in the streets with turntables. What started during that time as an underground subculture has emerged and evolved into something that is so much more than just music. Hip-hop has become a platform that incorporates art, fashion, politics, technology—you name it and there is a hip-hop song about it (chicken noodle soup with a soda on the side anyone?). Hip-hop has brought people together through all of these avenues, and ultimately that's what we are looking to do with fitness.

Mason and I also both love hip-hop. When we are at home hanging out, or doing dishes, or doing our own workouts, we are listening to hip-hop. It is music we truly love. That personal choice was a big part of what inspired us to fuse it with yoga. We had no idea if people would think we were

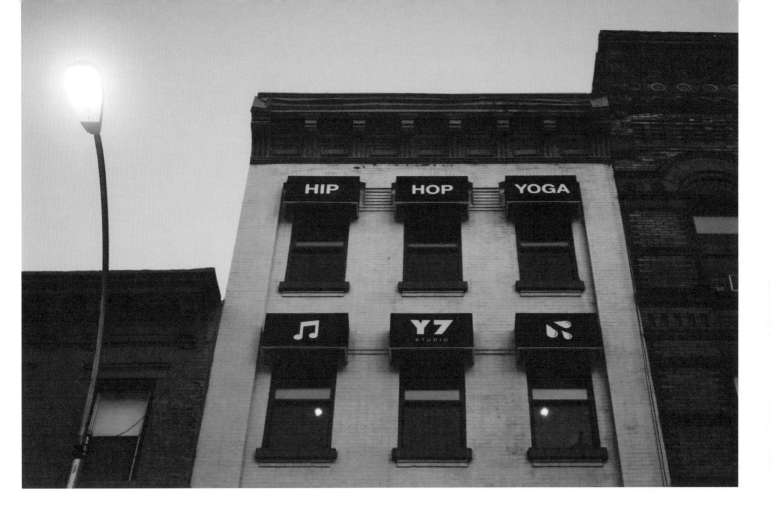

crazy or not. But think about this: when you are running on the treadmill, you start off slow for a warm-up and over time build up your pace to come to a peak before then cooling down. We wanted to evoke a similar feeling with yoga. The strong beat helps to drive your motivation and your desire to push yourself. That attitude of grit and determination is intrinsic to hip-hop—that feeling of always pushing yourself to be better. And, ultimately, that is a feeling ingrained in the culture of New York, the center of hip-hop's roots, as well. We found that the idea of being able to do yoga, which is so grounding and humbling, to sounds that are so inspiring and motivating was something that really resonated with people.

FINDING
YOUR BEATS

Music is at the heart of everything we do at Y7. The sequencing we create in our classes is crafted with music in mind: Which songs are relevant today? How are we linking breath to movement with the beat?

We use music to set the tone and create specific bursts of energy in class. Upon entering the dark, candlelit room, students are welcomed by soothing, slower beats, encouraging them to leave all of their stresses and worries at the door.

This intro is designed to get everyone to settle into the space. As we begin class, we slowly pump up the volume and increase the tempo of songs. This acceleration is meant to motivate, to encourage our clients to use their bodies to their fullest potential. The right song can motivate someone to hold that Chair Pose for just a little bit longer; pushing through those tough moments in class will ultimately enhance your practice and bring your body to a new level.

Traditionally, people practice yoga in silence, or music has been added as an afterthought to create ambience. At Y7, we bring music to the forefront, using it as an element in creating the experience. Picture walking into a 7:00 a.m. class: You're half asleep still and just thankful that you made it out of the apartment and to a fitness class so early. As you start the class, it is silent, just the instructor speaking and asking you to use this not-awake body to do difficult things. It's not so easy. What better way to make yoga accessible than to use a language we all understand—music?

Once you start allowing the music you love into your yoga practice, you'll see what a natural fit it is. The reasoning behind the pairing is so simple, but so powerful: just think about the way a baby reacts when she hears music, how she begins to move or smile or dance. The core of that reaction is the baby experiencing a change in mood in response to the music. Beginning in our earliest years, we respond to an innate connection between music and mood—the rhythms engage the brain and affect how we feel in ways both big and small. There's a reason why some of your most powerful memories are tied to songs and why movies always save their biggest musical numbers for the most important scenes.

We use music to motivate you to get that body moving, to challenge your mind and your physical self in those moments of doubt. We don't want you to take the easy road out and just drop into Child's Pose. We want you leaving class fulfilled, knowing that you gave it your all. When you are tired and you feel like you can't possibly hold your Plank for another ten breaths,

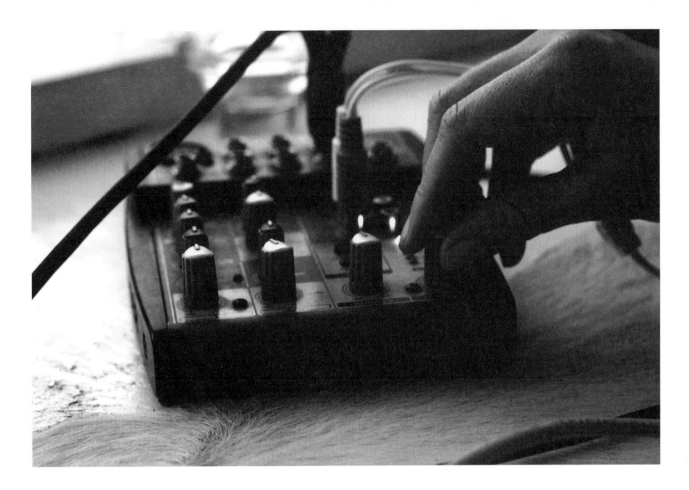

all it takes is that one song to keep you going. For so many of our students, when those moments come during class, the beat pumps them up and lets them know that they can make it through. Whether it's the beat, the lyrics, or just the mood, we make sure the driving force in the music becomes a driving force for our tribe as they push themselves to work just a little harder, to hold that pose a few more seconds, or to bend a little deeper. I love hip-hop music for that motivation—it has such a great variation of beats, and it's perfect for the one-breath-to-one-movement practice we offer in class and that you'll find in the sequences later in this book. (Don't worry, though—just because I love hip-hop, that doesn't mean you have to use that particular style of music to create a playlist that suits you!)

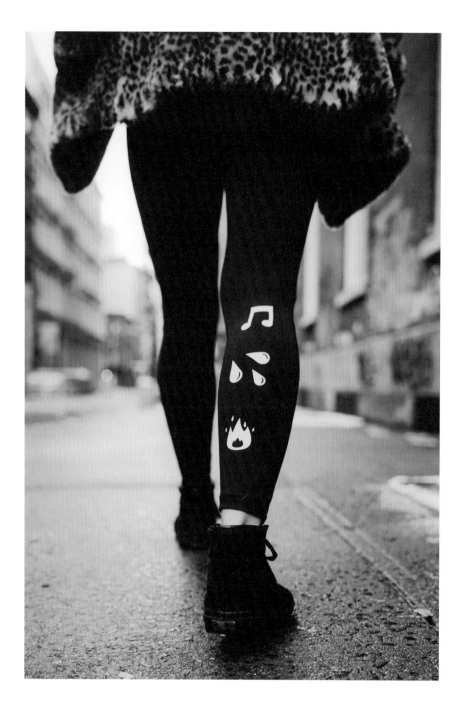

That's not to say music is only about propelling you through the hardest parts of your workout. Just like in life, music has a place in all parts of your yoga practice, from the fastest flow to the quiet satisfaction of the final Corpse Pose. At Y7, we use slower, more soothing music to help relax the mind and body at the end of class—it's important to give the body and mind time to come down from the heights of a strenuous class, and music is one of the best ways to make that transition. Put yourself in that situation: You have just worked your body and mind so hard, focusing on moving from pose to pose, keeping up with your breath, and concentrating on yourself. In the final section of your workout you should aim to let go of everything that just happened. Don't think about what you are doing after the workout, or what you could have done differently. Let go. Choosing the right music for this point in the sequence can get you to that centered place, full of peace of mind. For a lot of people this is the toughest part of the practice—we are always so eager to get on with our lives. But for even just one song, take the time to sit with yourself. Be in the present. These are the best moments in your yoga experience.

MAKING YOUR PLAYLIST

So you know that music is important, that music can bring your yoga practice to a completely different level, that music can make your workout your own. But how do you create that perfect playlist that matches your personality and your workout? First and foremost: *pick music that you love*. The music should motivate *you* and help you move the way you want to. At Y7 we prefer hip-hop (see page 36), but that doesn't mean you need to blast Tupac in your home in order to practice (though we highly recommend it).

If you are not feeling hip-hop for your flow, rest assured that there are plenty of options for you. When I am looking for something different for my flows, one of my favorite things to do is look at music apps (like Spotify or Pandora) to get inspired. Search for chill hits, dance, or rhythmic beats; see how these different options make you feel. When I practice, I like to either feel a calming vibe (if I want a more relaxed workout) or something super upbeat (if I am tired but really want to work). The kind of music you choose can really change your attitude. So if you are unmotivated, pick music that will lift you up. And remember, music can influence you in a lot of different ways: when you are settling onto your mat or cooling down, you want to clear your mind, so for those periods I suggest avoiding music with lyrics that can trigger any anxiety or frustration. You want to be able to leave all of your feelings and attachments about your practice on the mat.

At the studio we try to keep things fresh and fun by allowing our instructors to pick music themes based on their personal preferences. We have done a whole range from one-hit wonders or boy bands to '90s hip-hop, emerging artists, and even battle classes between two feuding artists. One of my absolute favorite themes is Jock Jams. (I am pretty sure this dates me.)

Consider picking themes for your own workouts, especially if you're organizing a group practice—it can add a completely new, fun dimension to the session.

Besides choosing the type of music you want, you also need to decide what kind of flow you want to do. There are a few questions that can help you determine your flow:

DO YOU WANT ··········· **SOMETHING RESTORATIVE AND SLOW OR MORE FAST-PACED AND UPBEAT?**

DO YOU WANT ··········· **A FULL, HOURLONG, CLASS-LENGTH SEQUENCE OR SOMETHING THAT'S MORE CONDENSED?**

DO YOU WANT ··········· **THE SAME MOOD THROUGHOUT YOUR ENTIRE WORKOUT, OR DO YOU WANT TO VARY THE MOOD?**

DO YOU WANT ··········· **TO PUSH YOUR LIMITS IN TERMS OF POSES, OR DO YOU WANT TO WORK MORE WITHIN YOUR COMFORT ZONE?**

Your answers to these questions will dictate the pace of your playlist. There are also certain basic principles that I always like to keep in mind when crafting a music sequence in the studio. Each section of the workout will last a certain amount of time, which will correspond to the number of songs needed and the number of poses you'll flow through. It's also helpful to consider how intense each segment of the workout will be, both for you physically and in terms of the music you're playing (at Y7, we sync this up with the music's beats per minute, or bpm).

Below you'll find two charts that I've developed to guide our choices as we build our flows and our playlists. Don't think of these as a set of rules you have to adhere to, but instead as jumping-off points for finding the match between postures and music that works for you.

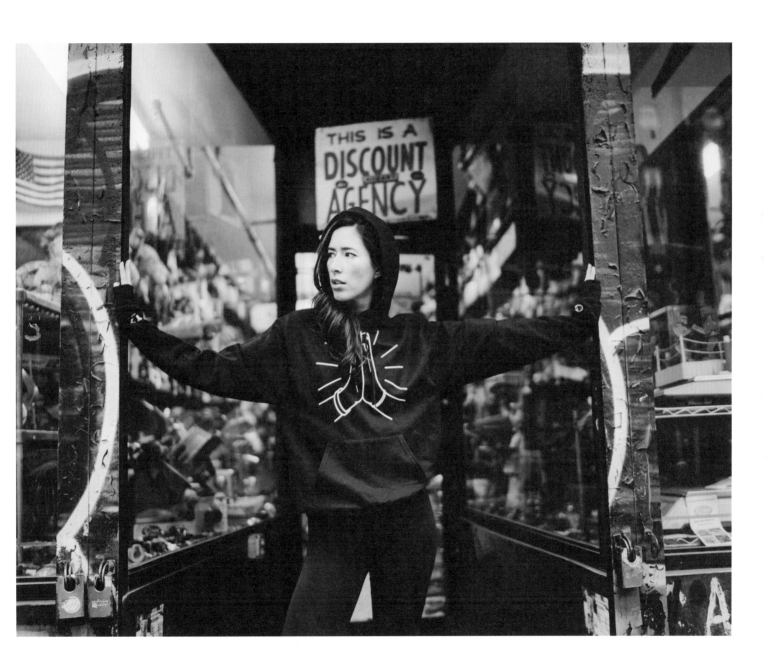

Flow Guidelines

	LENGTH/ DURATION	POSTURE GUIDELINES
SETTLE IN/ WARM-UP	Under 10 minutes total	Shapes that warm and open the body: Child's Pose, Cat & Cow, Down Dog, spinal twists, Staff Pose prep
FLOW 1	3 postures (not including Down Dog, Sun Salutation A, Upward Salute)	Warm-up shapes + Sun Salutation A, Upward Salute, Low Lunge Twist, Low Crescent Lunge or hamstring stretches and side bends
FLOW 2	7 postures	Primarily warrior shapes: W1, W2, Side Angle, Triangle, Side Plank, Half Moon, Chair, Crow
FLOW 3	8 postures	High-energy peak postures: High Lunge, W3, Eagle, Hand-to-Big Toe, Chair, Handstand, Forearm Stand, arm balances
CHILD'S POSE	2 minutes	Child's Pose with an option of Headstand
SLOW BURN	3 minutes with each posture being held for 1 minute each side	Shapes that generate a muscular burn: Chair, High Lunge, Plank, Boat, Locust, Bridge/Wheel (e.g., High Lunge 1 minute each side and Plank 1 minute)
RESTORATIVE	3 postures	Shapes that restore: Pigeon, Plow, Shoulder Stand, Reclined Twist, Happy Baby
CORPSE POSE	3 minutes	Corpse

Music Guidelines

	SONG CHOICE	TIME FRAME	POSTURE GUIDELINES
SETTLE IN/ WARM-UP	Instrumental song with soft tempo and no bass	Under 10 minutes	Poses that warm up the body: Child's Pose, Cat & Cow, Down Dog, side bends
FLOW 1	Low tempo electronic/hip-hop with a beat (100–110 bpm)	10 minutes	Sun Salutations, Upward Salute, Low Lunge, half splits
FLOW 2	Moderate tempo electronic/ hip-hop/ pop/R&B (120–130 bpm)	10 minutes	Standing poses: W1, W2, Triangle, Half Moon, Chair
FLOW 3	Highest energy, most motivating, strongest lyrical hip-hop/ electronic/pop (135–145 bpm)	12 minutes	Balancing poses: High Lunge, Twisted High Lunge, W3, Eagle, Forearm Stand, arm balances
COOLDOWN	Can be instrumental music with moderate tempo	3 minutes	Child's Pose/Goddess Pose
RESTORATIVE	Relaxing music with little to no beat	10 minutes	Pigeon, Plow, Shoulder Stand, Reclined Twist, Happy Baby
CORPSE POSE	Instrumental music with no beat and no lyrics—setting the tone for students to meditate and go inside	3 minutes	Corpse Pose

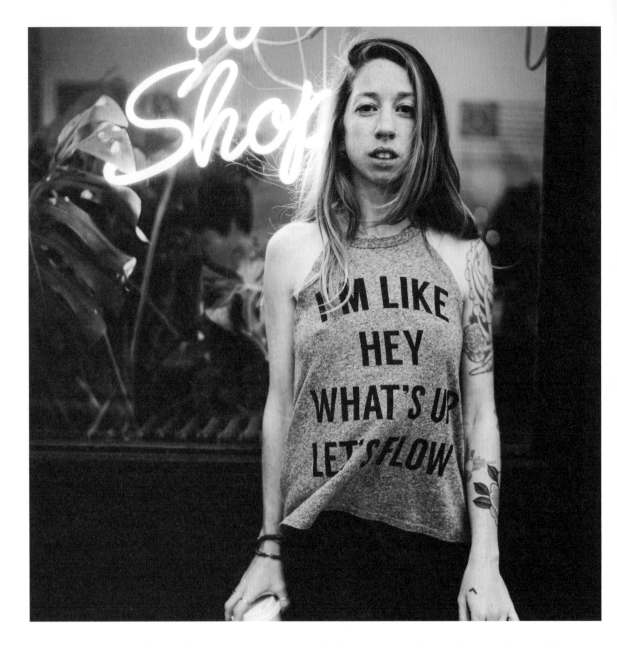

Now we'll go over the principles for the two main types of workouts in a little more depth: a fast-paced flow and a calming sequence. Once you've got the basics for these down, you'll be able to adapt the ideas to any workout.

Vinyasa Flow

When you choose to do an intense, heat-building flow, you'll want to think of the music as an arc, with a peak at the top that then drops down to your cooldown phase. In general, this kind of flow can be broken down into:

OPENING/WARM-UP ·········· **5–8 MINUTES (1–2 SONGS)**
EXAMPLE ARTISTS: THE XX, FKA TWIGS, BANKS

SONGS BUILDING IN INTENSITY ·········· **20 MINUTES (4–5 SONGS)**
EXAMPLE ARTISTS: THE WEEKND, MIGUEL, BEYONCÉ

PEAK ·········· **10–12 MINUTES (3–4 SONGS)**
EXAMPLE ARTISTS: CALVIN HARRIS, A$AP ROCKY, MAJOR LAZER, J. COLE

COOLDOWN ·········· **5–8 MINUTES (1–2 SONGS)**
EXAMPLE ARTISTS: JHENÉ AIKO, FRANK OCEAN

Here's an example of a playlist that will work for a fast-paced flow. It highlights the type of music you'd hear at a typical Y7 class, and it's perfect for a workout that lasts about fifty minutes.

VINYASA FLOW PLAYLIST

"Love for That" by Mura Masa (3:09)

"The Morning" by the Weeknd (5:12)

"Simple Things (remix)" by Miguel (3:58)

"What's My Name" by Rihanna (4:22)

"Beggin for Thread" by Banks (4:10)

"Power Trip" by J. Cole (4:00)

"Beware" by Big Sean (3:57)

"Don't Tell 'Em" by Jeremih (4:27)

"10 Bands" by Drake (2:58)

"Carry Out" by Timbaland (3:59)

"The Vapors" by Jhené Aiko (3:31)

"The Place" by Inc. (3:41)

"Missing Photos" by Last Days (2:04)

Restorative Flow

If you are doing a more restorative practice, your focus won't be on the high-energy flow that characterizes vinyasa. Instead, you'll be working on stretching your muscles and deepening your poses, so it is better to have a more consistent beat throughout your playlist that you can cue your breath with. When crafting a music sequence for your restorative flow, emphasize songs that make you feel grounded and calm. If any song induces any anxiety, you should probably take it out—stressful emotions won't serve you in a more mindful practice. When practicing restorative yoga, I like to focus on the breathing pattern of a five-count inhale and a seven-count exhale. All of the songs you pick for this kind of playlist should be below 120 bpm, to avoid triggering fast movements that will increase your heart rate. Some artists to look at are: The xx, Inc. No World, FKA Twigs, AU, Sigur Rós, and Bon Iver.

This example playlist will work well for a restorative flow lasting about fifty minutes.

RESTORATIVE FLOW PLAYLIST

"Remi (Essay Remix)" by Kyson (6:35)

"Nitesky" by Robot Koch (4:41)

"Twice (Aaron Jerome Remix)"
   by Little Dragon (5:00)

"Lay Your Cards Out" by Polica (4:05)

"Afterglow" by Phaeleh (4:43)

"Water Me" by FKA Twigs (3:30)

"Rescue Song (RAC Remix)"
   by Mr. Little Jeans (4:16)

"Boute" by AU (4:07)

"Desert Rose" by Inc. (3:54)

"Too Much" by Sampha (2:57)

"Goat Mountain" by Loscil (10:30)

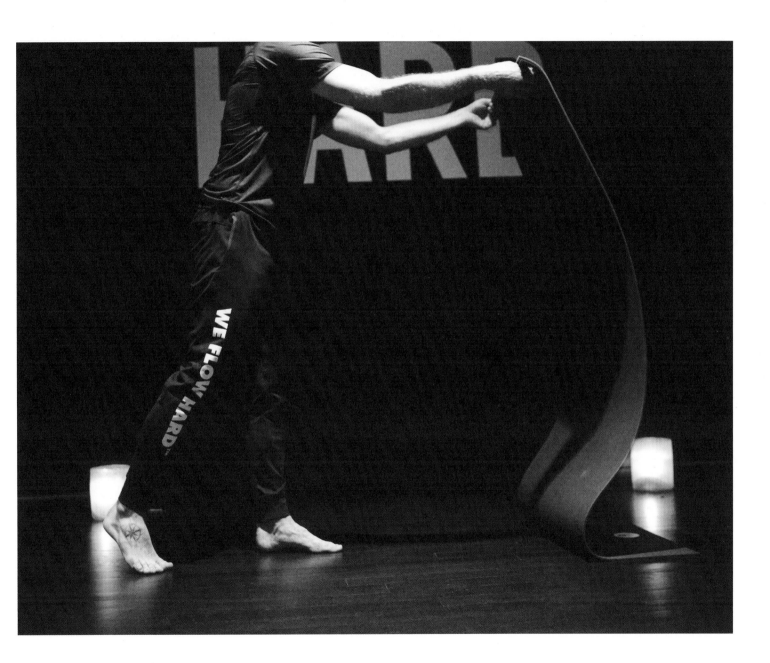

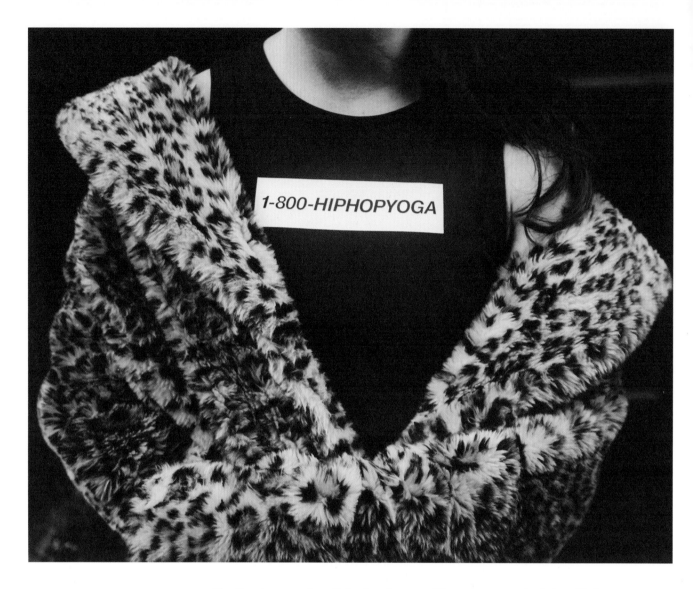

You'll get so much satisfaction from crafting your own playlists with the music that you love best—there's nothing like flowing along to beats that have personal meaning for you. But there's also something great about having some playlists ready to go whenever you need them! So we've also created one to go along with each of the sequences in the next section to get you started. Namaste.

WARM-UP SEQUENCE (SEE PAGE 58)

"Slide" by Calvin Harris (3:50)

"Run Up" by Major Lazer (3:23)

"Wyclef Jean" by Young Thug (3:56)

"X" by 21 Savage (4:19)

"Imma Star" by Jeremih (4:21)

"Fashion Killa" by A$AP Rocky (3:56)

"Never Forget You" by Zara Larsson (3:33)

"Right Now" by Akon (4:01)

Y7 FLOW (SEE PAGE 76)

"Sunburn" by Tinashe (3:59)

"Money Trees" by Kendrick Lamar (6:26)

"Turnin' Me Up" by BJ The Chicago Kid (4:29)

"Get Money" by The Notorious B.I.G. (4:34)

"I Like Tuh" by Carnage (3:07)

"Why You Always Hatin?" by YG, Drake, Kamaiyah (3:16)

"Who Run It" by Three 6 Mafia (4:09)

Y7 MEGA DETOX (SEE PAGE 96)

"Shouldn't Have Done That" by Two Another (4:25)

"Best to You" by Blood Orange (3:45)

"Suede Jaw" by 808INK (2:23)

"Slide" by Calvin Harris, Frank Ocean, Migos (3:50)

"By Design" by Kid Cudi, Andre Benjamin (4:17)

"Get By" by Talib Kweli (3:47)

"Love Somebody" by Ta-ku Wafia (3:28)

ABS & ASS SEQUENCE (SEE PAGE 112)

"I'm Better" by Missy Elliott (3:33)

"A Tale of 2 Citiez" by J. Cole (4:30)

"Bad and Boujee" by Migos (5:43)

"Countdown" by Beyoncé (3:32)

"Feeling Myself" by Nicki Minaj (3:58)

"No Scrubs" by TLC (3:34)

"You Know What It Is" by T.I. (4:47)

"Swang" by Rae Sremmurd (3:28)

STRIKE
A POSE

Yoga, especially at Y7, is all about your individual experience, what you bring to the mat. There are the preparations you do beforehand, from deciding on the goals for your practice to picking the perfect beats. And then there are the poses, which make up the core of your physical experience. At our studios we focus on two main types of sequences—fast-paced vinyasa flows make up our We Flow Hard classes, while our Slow Burn classes feature more restorative flows that allow you to go deeper into the poses.

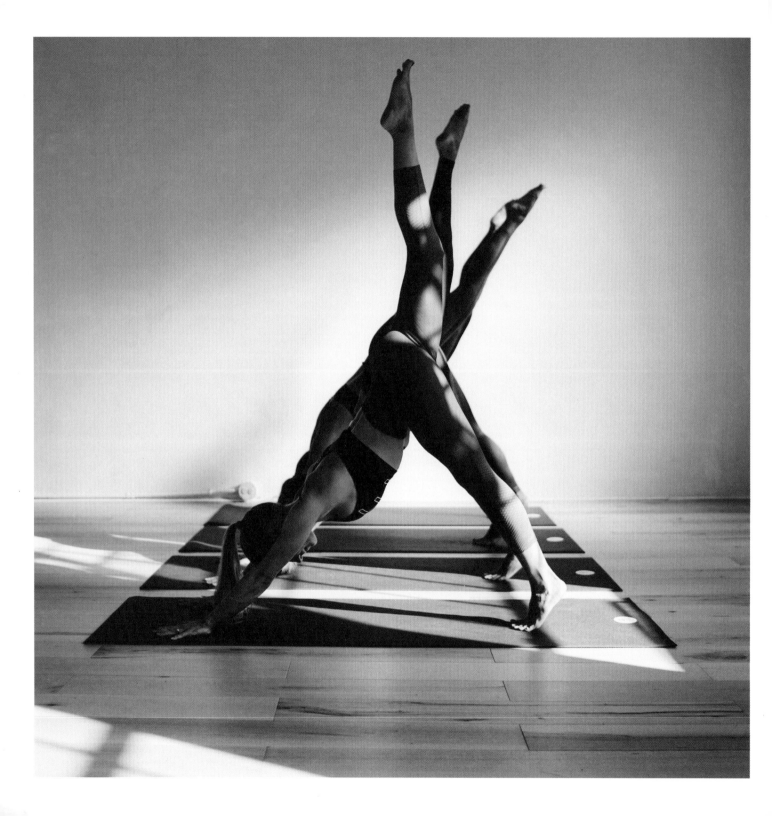

Vinyasa is mindful, flowing movement. In vinyasa, we move through postures with intention, braiding poses together that open, stretch, and restore the body from the inside out. In the coming sequences you'll work to link breath and movement and bring a greater consciousness to the connection between mind and body. The transformative movement in these flows is meant to push you—to explore and move past what you believe your limits to be in a smart, safe way. We've included a variety of sequences that incorporate a fast, invigorating pace from a signature Y7 Flow to a more intense Major Detox and a targeted Abs & Ass Sequence.

In our studios, the Slow Burn works toward not only reaching our edge, but surpassing it. These classes guide you deeper and deeper into a carefully selected series of postures, with the attentive assistance of an instructor. In this book, you'll find a similar feeling in the Warm-Up sequence, which focuses on foundation and structure within our movement. You'll be asked to place emphasis on both the necessity and support our breath allots us as practitioners, using pranayama to both inspire our movement and guide our mind. This type of flow can be equally beneficial as a warm-up to a more intense cardio workout or as a way to unplug and tune in to your body's essential rhythms after a long day.

The sequences here were developed by our Y7 artists—instructors who love to bring challenging, fun yoga to our students. Their perspectives are a key part of what we do at Y7, and their individual voices are felt in the flows they've contributed—the sequences aren't all one way, because our classes aren't all taught the same way. As you try these flows, enter the space they've created and cast aside the expectations you carry every day. Come to the mat with an open mind, prepared to sweat, work, breathe, and restore yourself.

As you build your practice, your newfound agility will be balanced by strength, coordination, and enhanced cardiovascular health, as well as a sense of physical confidence and overall well-being.

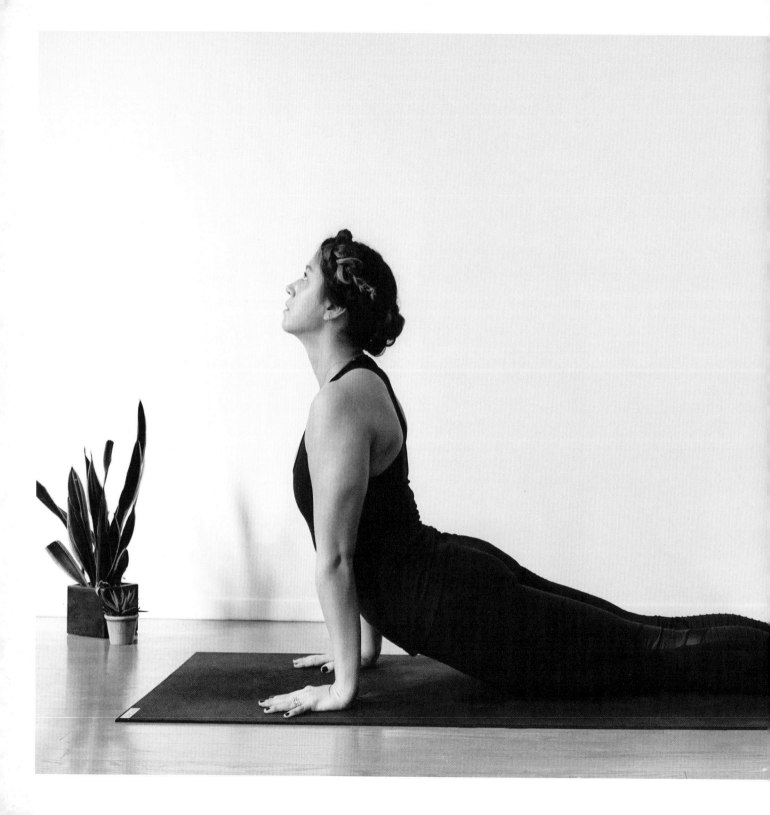

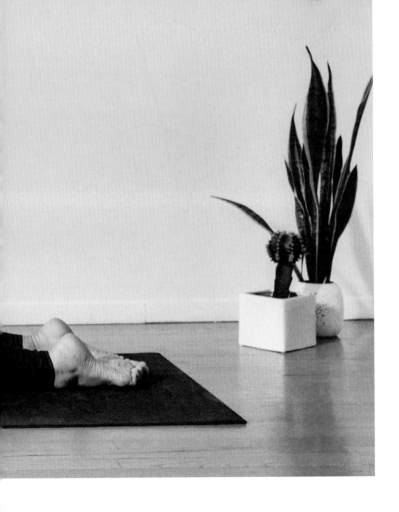

Warm-Up Sequence

(SARAH L.)

Sarah is the cofounder of Y7 Studio and a 200-hour Registered Yoga Teacher (RYT).

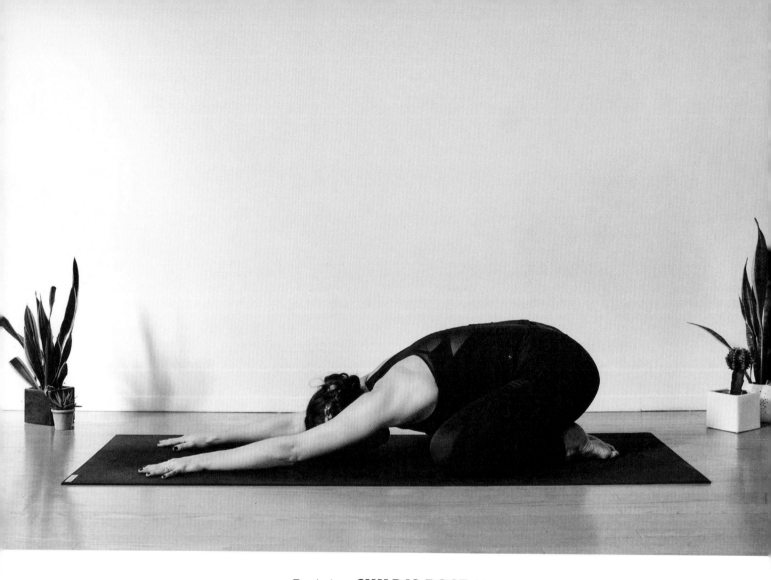

Begin in a **CHILD'S POSE**. Keep your toes together, knees spread wide apart, as your chest melts down between your legs. Your arms will stretch out long in front of you. Take a big breath in and a big breath out.

On your next inhale rise up onto your hands and knees into a **TABLETOP** position. Your hands and knees should be firmly planted into the mat, your shoulders directly over your wrists. Your neck will be long and your gaze should be right in front of your fingertips. Suck the belly into the spine, creating a long line of energy with a neutral spine. Stay here for a full breath (inhale and exhale).

On an inhale, arch your spine and bring your gaze to the sky for **COW POSE**.

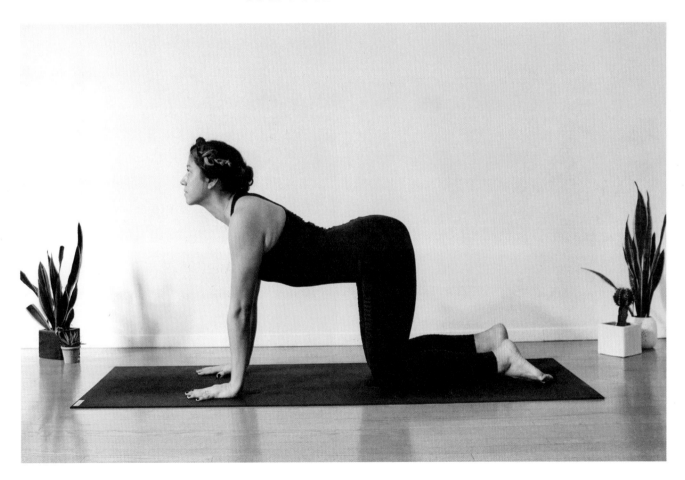

On your exhale, round your back as you drop your head and look toward your belly button, coming into **CAT POSE**.

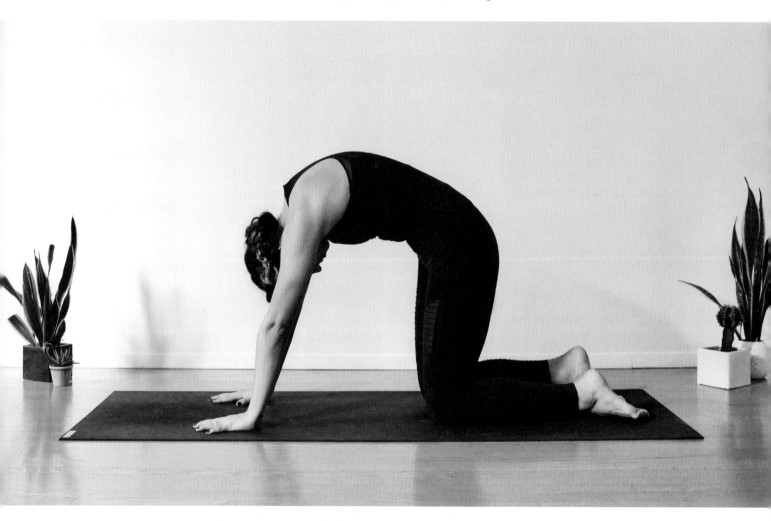

Moving with your breath, begin three rounds of **CAT** and **COW**, warming up the spine. Consider making these movements your own by swiveling the hips or flipping the palms.

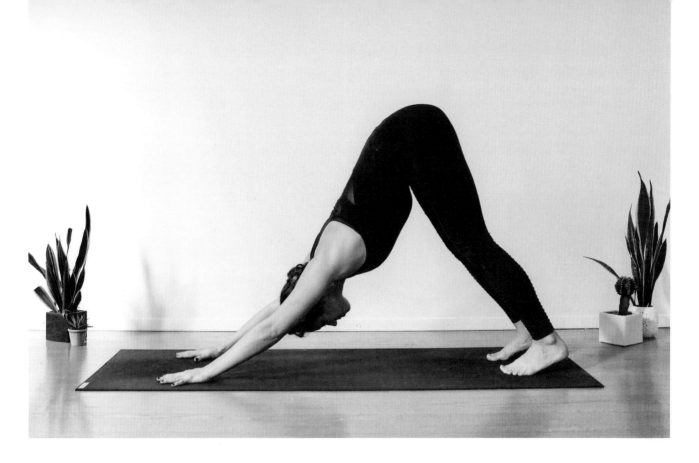

When you have finished your third full breath, tuck your toes and lift your hips into **DOWNWARD FACING DOG**. Once you arrive there, spread your fingertips wide, making sure your thumb and first finger are firmly planted in the ground—holding a bit more weight than the rest of the hand. Your biceps should be rotating toward the ears, so the inner part of your elbow is facing the front of the room. Activate the inner thighs as you lift the hips farther toward the sky. Your feet should be hip's width apart and parallel to one another, with toes pointed to the front of the mat as your heels reach toward the ground. If you choose, stay here for a few cycles of breaths.

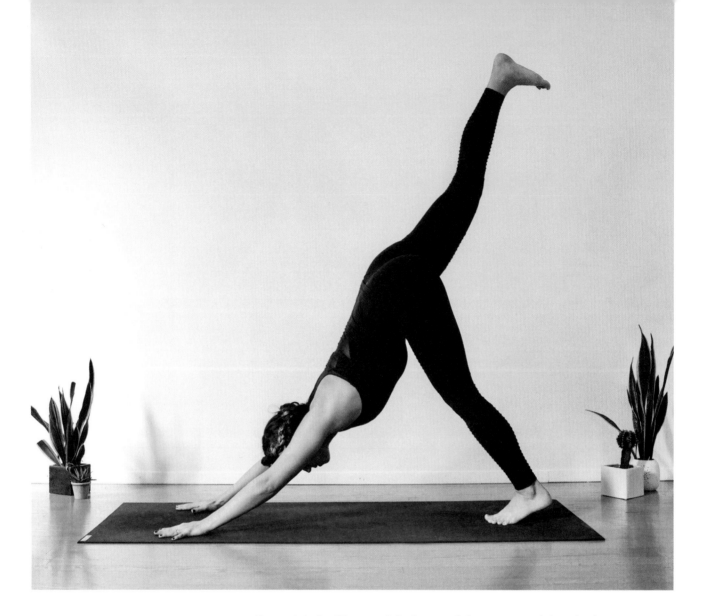

On an inhale, lift your right leg straight up toward the sky into a
DOWNWARD DOG SPLIT.

On your exhale step your foot forward into a **LOW LUNGE**, keeping the fingertips on the ground—your foot should land in between your hands. Bring your gaze in front of the fingers as you stay here for a full breath.

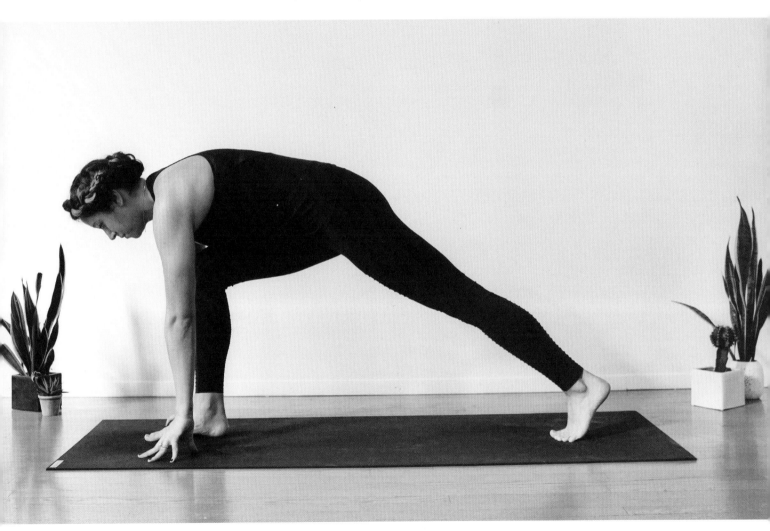

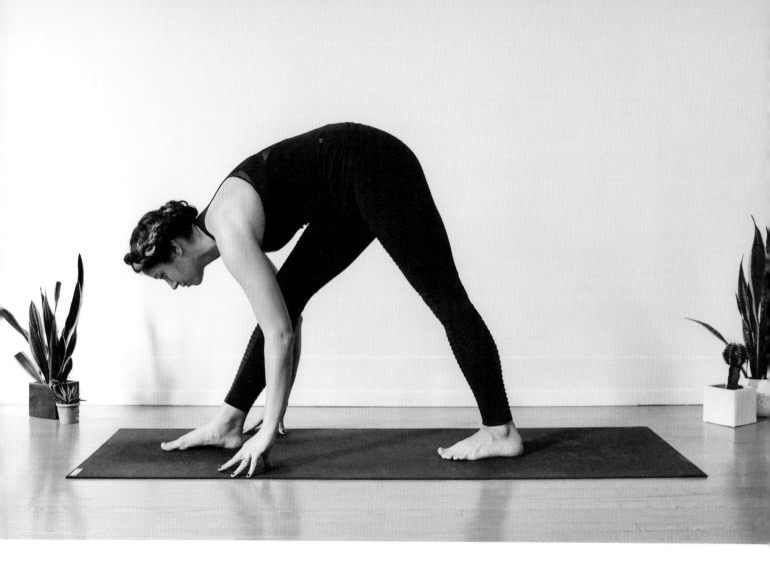

When you finish your exhale, begin to tuck your toes, keeping your
back leg long as you straighten the front leg as much as you can,
coming into **PYRAMID POSE**. Keep your chest draped over the
front leg—your forehead may touch your leg. If you are having trouble
or this pose is challenging for you, step your back leg in as much as
you need to in order to feel stable and grounded.

On an exhale, step your left foot to meet your right coming into a **FORWARD FOLD**. Let your head hang, relaxing the neck. You may want to reach your hands for your opposite elbows, or bring the hands interlaced behind the head for a deeper stretch.

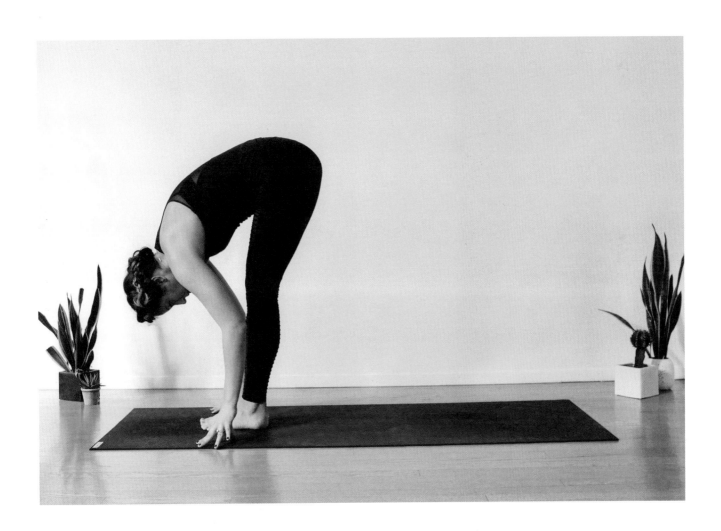

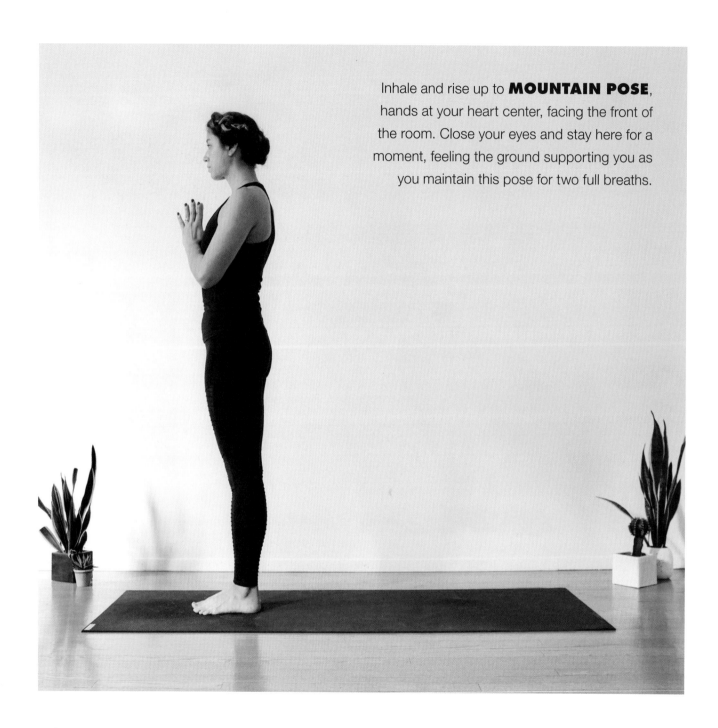

Inhale and rise up to **MOUNTAIN POSE**, hands at your heart center, facing the front of the room. Close your eyes and stay here for a moment, feeling the ground supporting you as you maintain this pose for two full breaths.

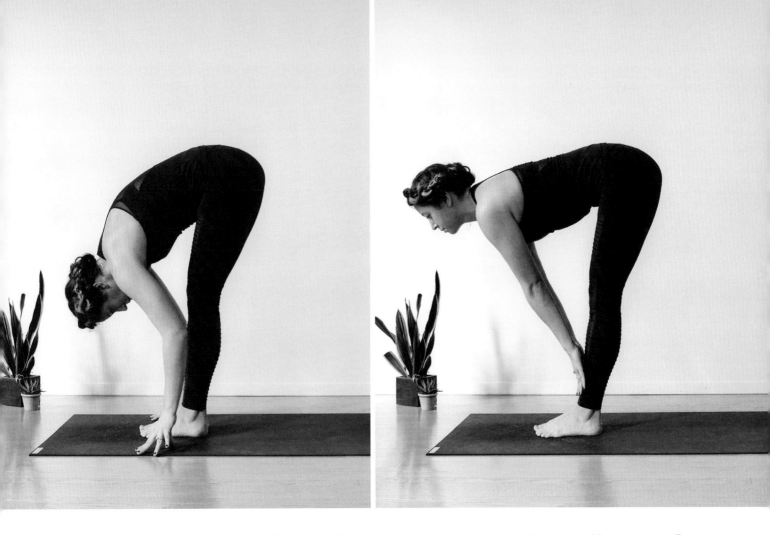

Take a big inhale, and as you exhale move from your hips to swan dive your arms down to the mat, coming back into a **FORWARD FOLD**.

As you inhale, bring your hands to your shins and look up, keeping a flat back, coming into a **HALFWAY LIFT**.

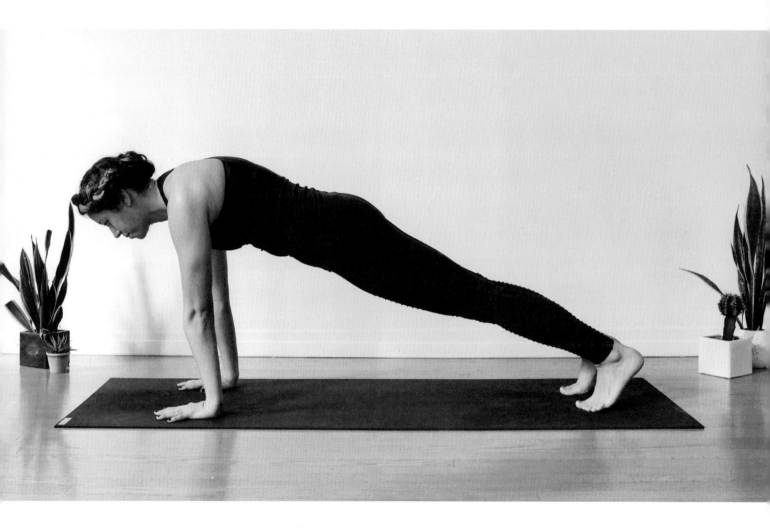

Bring both hands down to the ground and step back to a
PLANK POSE. Your shoulders should be directly over your wrists.
Extend your heels back and pull up through the thighs, reaching the
tailbone back to create one long line with your body. Stay here for
three full breaths, firing up the core.

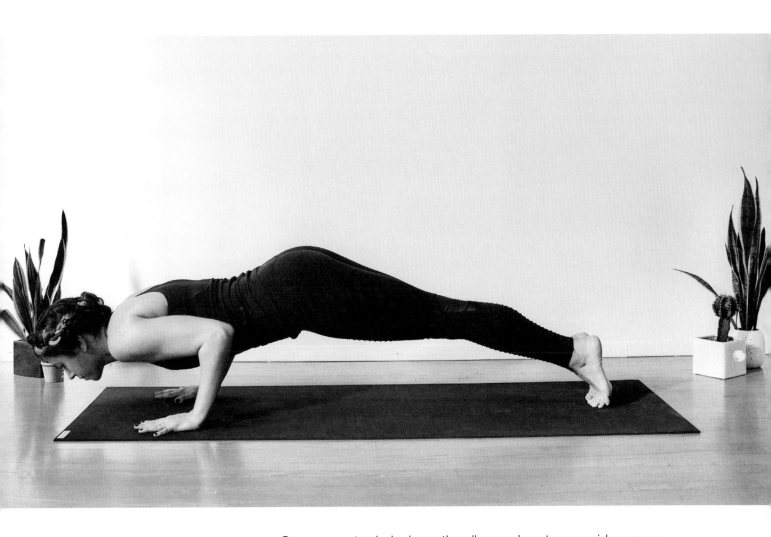

On your next exhale, keep the elbows close to your sides as you lower halfway down into **CHATURANGA DANDASANA**, also known as **STAFF POSE**—in this pose, your elbows should be bent to a 90-degree angle.

Inhale, flip the toes, and press the chest forward and up, gliding through to **UPWARD FACING DOG**. Only your hands and the tops of the feet should be on the ground, your thighs and knees should be active and lifted.

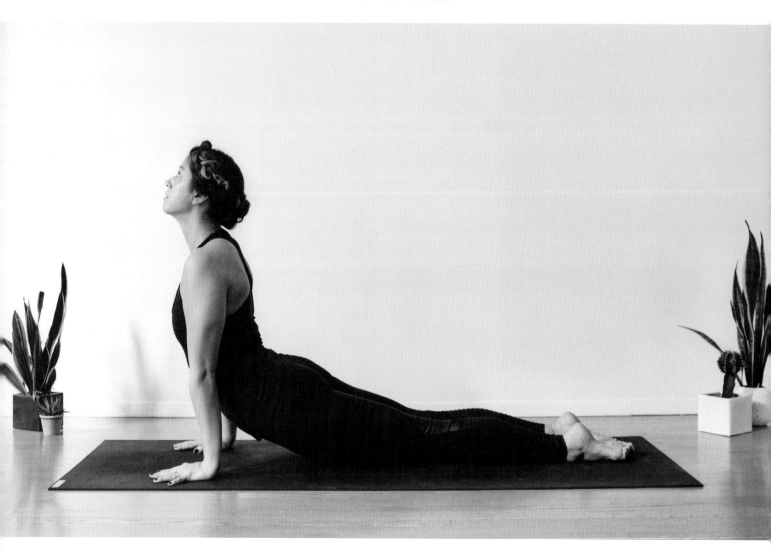

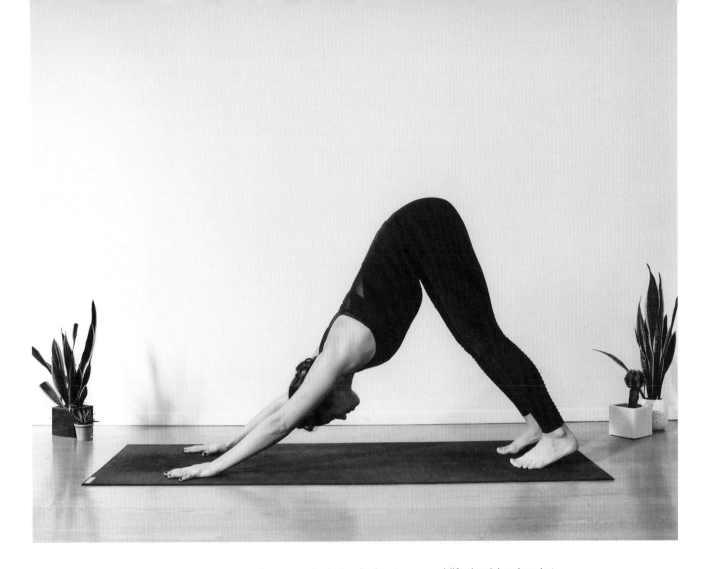

On an exhale tuck the toes and lift the hips back to
DOWNWARD FACING DOG.

Repeat the full sequence on your left side.

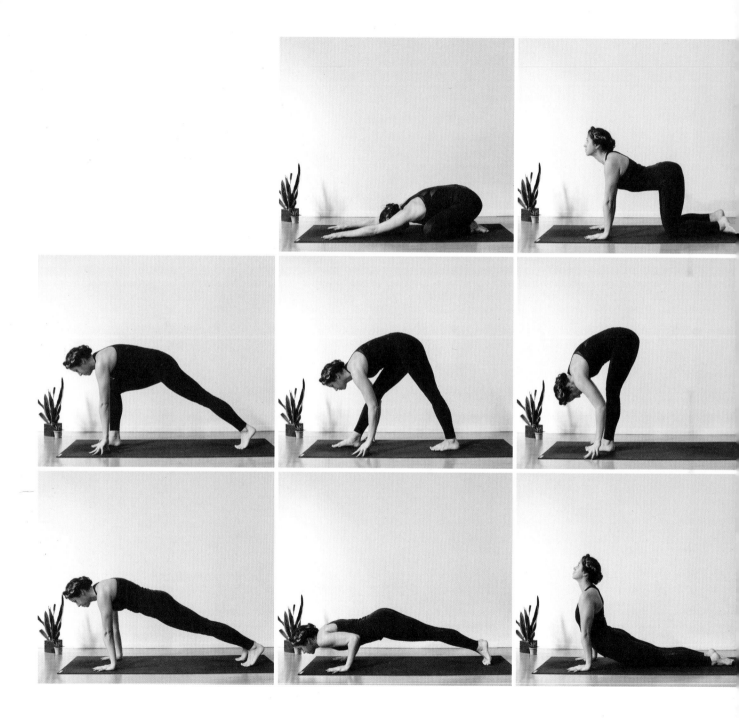

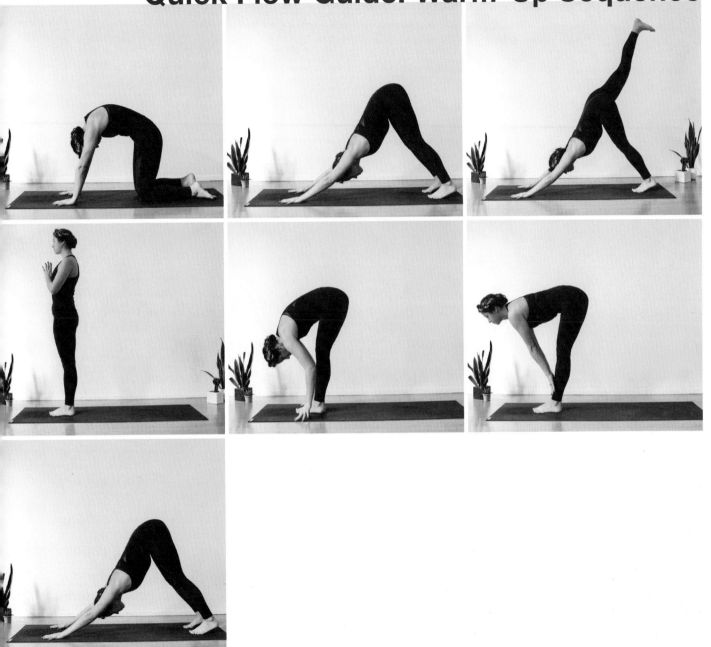

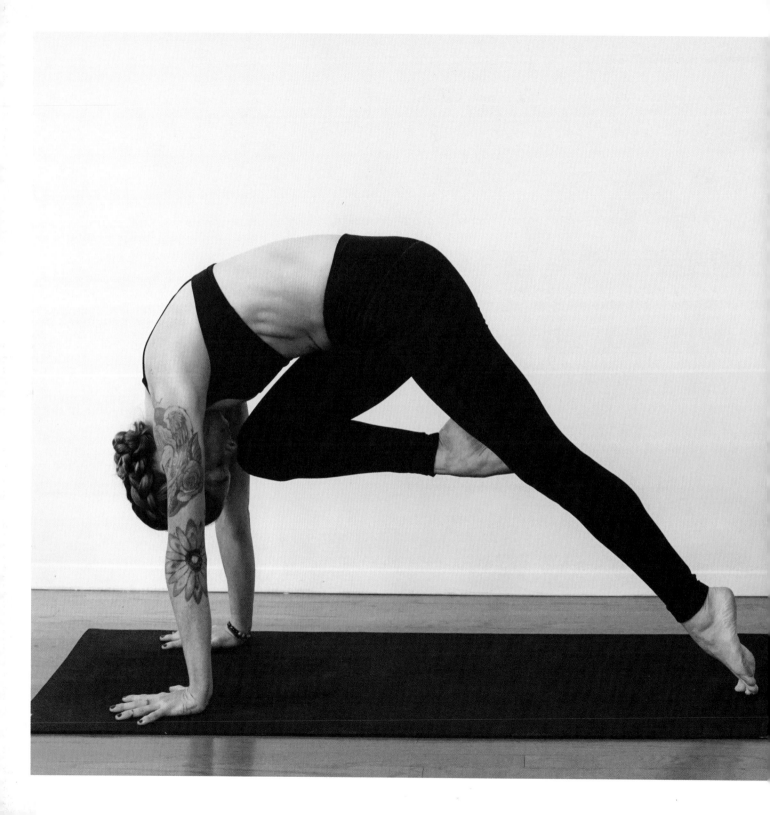

Y7 Flow

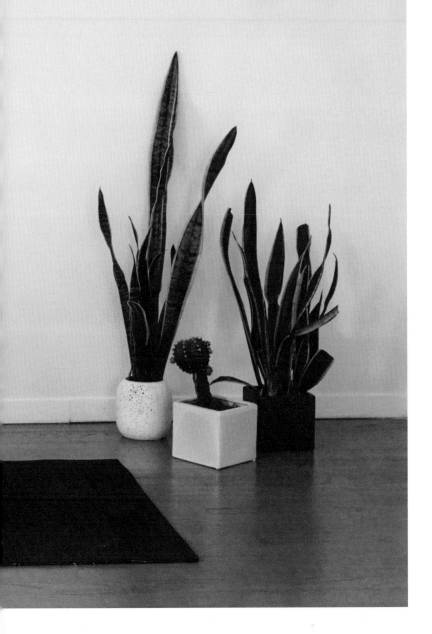

(KRISTEN N.)

Kristen is a 500-hour Experienced Registered Yoga Teacher (ERYT) and one of the 200-hour Yoga Teacher Training leaders for Y7.

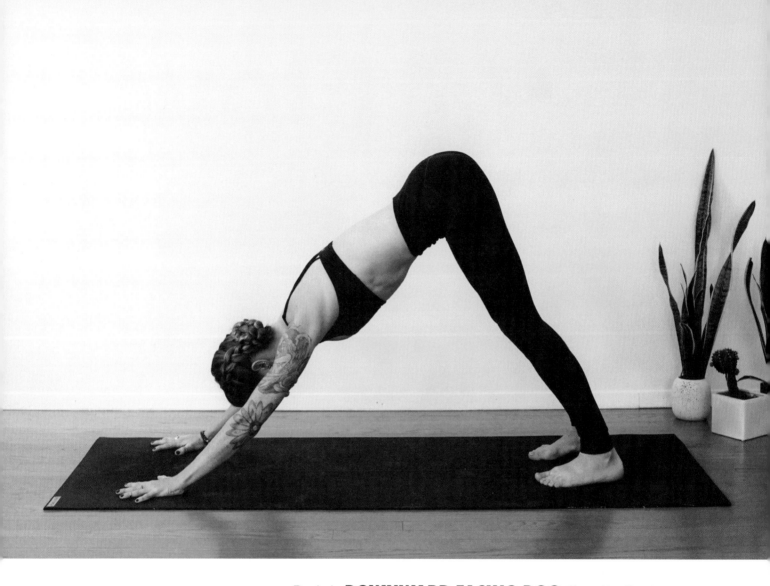

Begin in **DOWNWARD FACING DOG**. Pay attention to your breath here, and create a rhythmic pattern by finding an equal inhale and exhale.

After a few full breaths, inhale as you shift your weight forward into **PLANK POSE**. Be mindful that you align your shoulders on top of your wrists and do not lock your elbows. Keep your shoulders and hips in a straight line, as if the body is a board.

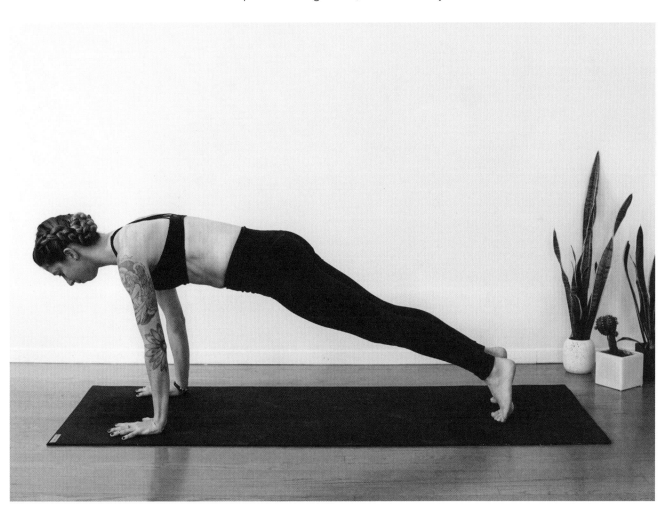

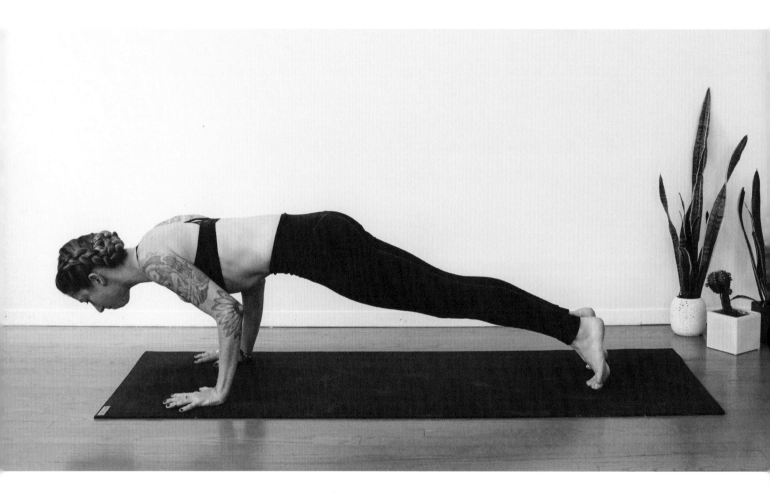

Breathe out and begin to lower the body halfway to the ground into **CHATURANGA DANDASANA**. Keep your elbows hugged into the body and make sure they are bent no more than 90 degrees.

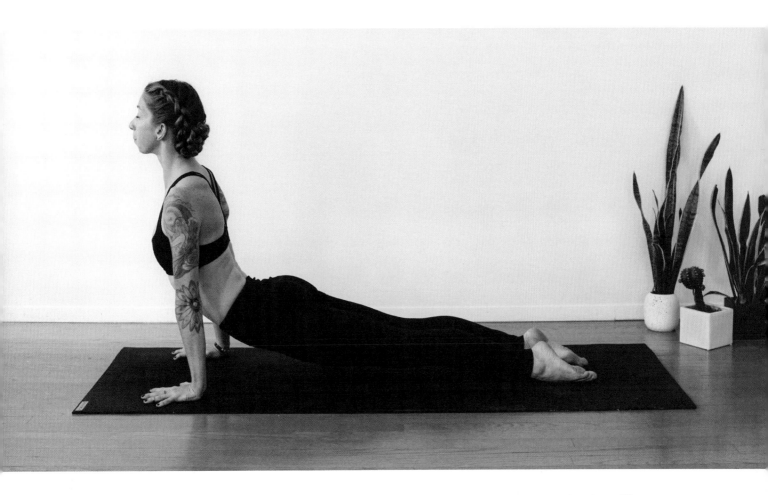

Inhale and press your hands into the floor as you begin to lift your chest forward and up, straightening out your arms and coming into **UPWARD FACING DOG**. Keep only your hands and feet on the ground as you activate your legs, core, and back muscles.

Exhale, lifting your hips back and up into **DOWNWARD FACING DOG**. Spread your fingertips wide, applying slightly more pressure at the thumb and index finger. Wrap your triceps in toward your armpits.

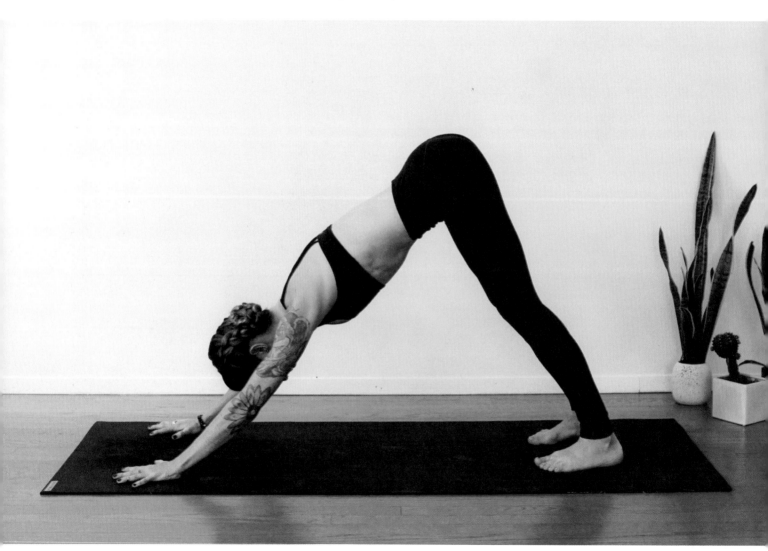

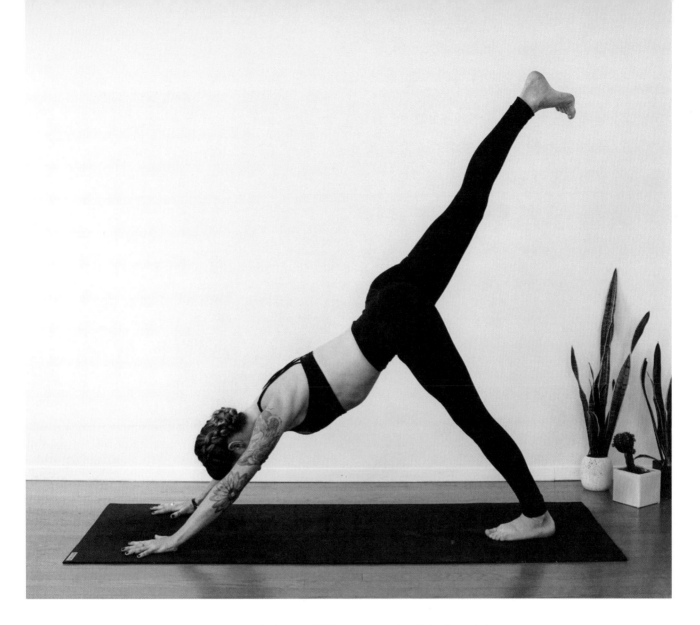

Inhale, and lift your right leg into the air into a
DOWNWARD DOG SPLIT, keeping your hips in one line.
Exhale, draw your knee to meet your nose, rounding your spine
and engaging the abdominal wall.

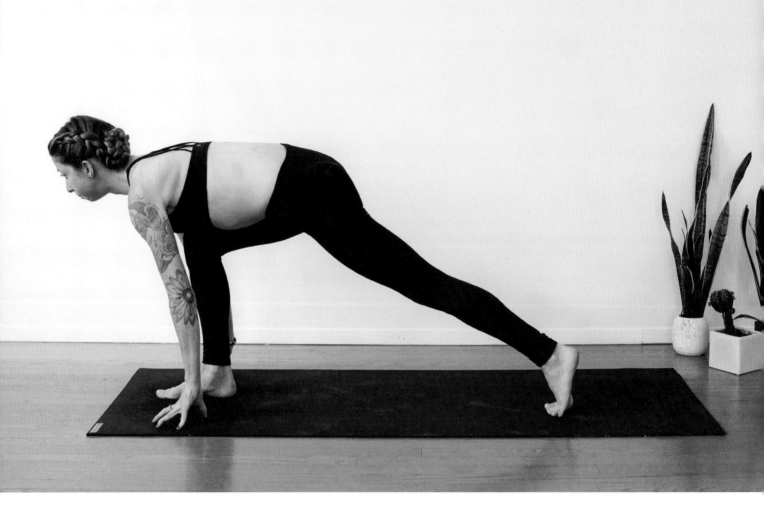

Keeping your core engaged, step your foot between your hands as lightly as you can into a **LOW LUNGE**.

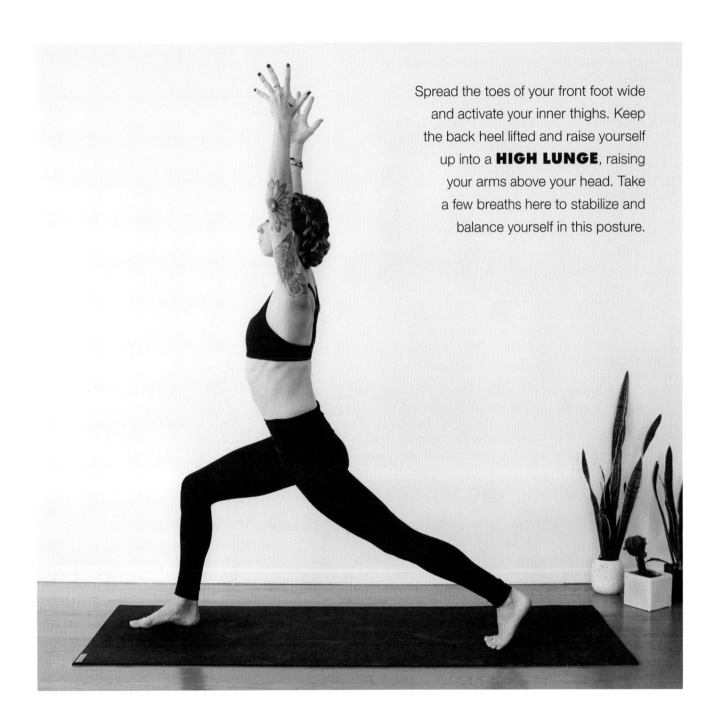

Spread the toes of your front foot wide and activate your inner thighs. Keep the back heel lifted and raise yourself up into a **HIGH LUNGE**, raising your arms above your head. Take a few breaths here to stabilize and balance yourself in this posture.

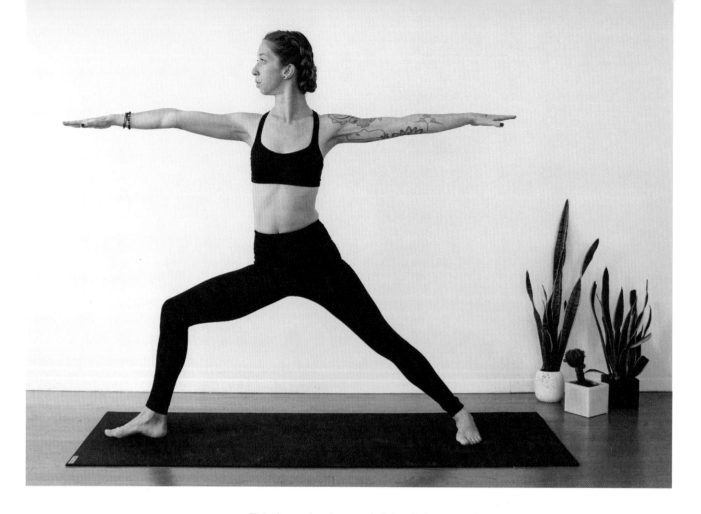

Exhale and spin your left heel down to the ground, opening your arms and hips to the side of your mat for **WARRIOR TWO**. Check out your front knee at this point—stack it on top of your ankle and line the knee up with your second toe. Engage your inner thighs by squeezing your heels in toward each other. Hold this pose for three to five breath cycles.

Maintain the base of your body and flip your right palm to face the ceiling, coming into **REVERSE WARRIOR** by reaching toward the back of the room and finding length in the right side body without collapsing into the left side body.

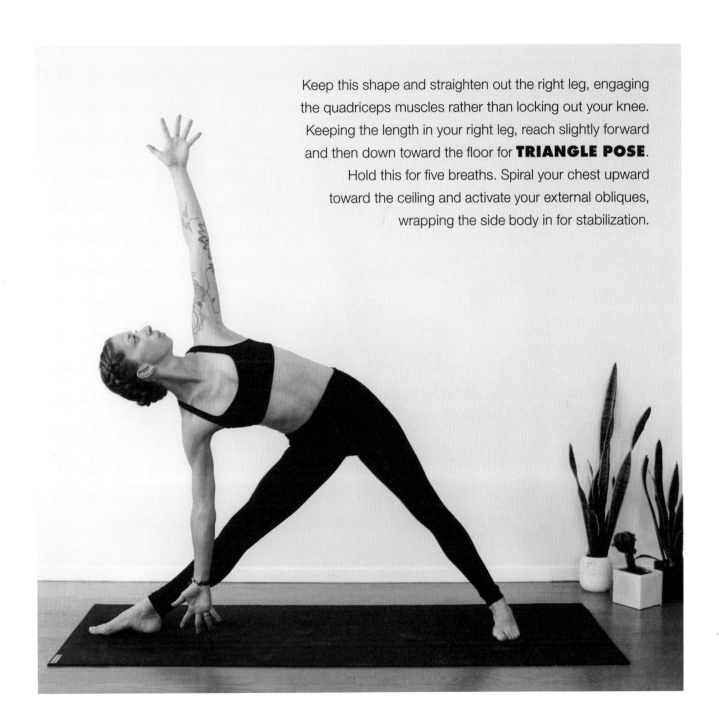

Keep this shape and straighten out the right leg, engaging the quadriceps muscles rather than locking out your knee. Keeping the length in your right leg, reach slightly forward and then down toward the floor for **TRIANGLE POSE**. Hold this for five breaths. Spiral your chest upward toward the ceiling and activate your external obliques, wrapping the side body in for stabilization.

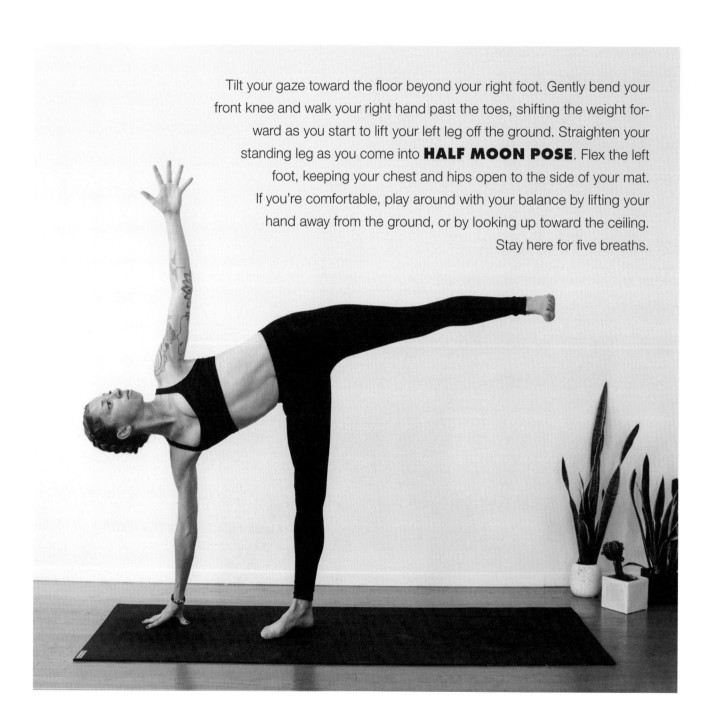

Tilt your gaze toward the floor beyond your right foot. Gently bend your front knee and walk your right hand past the toes, shifting the weight forward as you start to lift your left leg off the ground. Straighten your standing leg as you come into **HALF MOON POSE**. Flex the left foot, keeping your chest and hips open to the side of your mat. If you're comfortable, play around with your balance by lifting your hand away from the ground, or by looking up toward the ceiling. Stay here for five breaths.

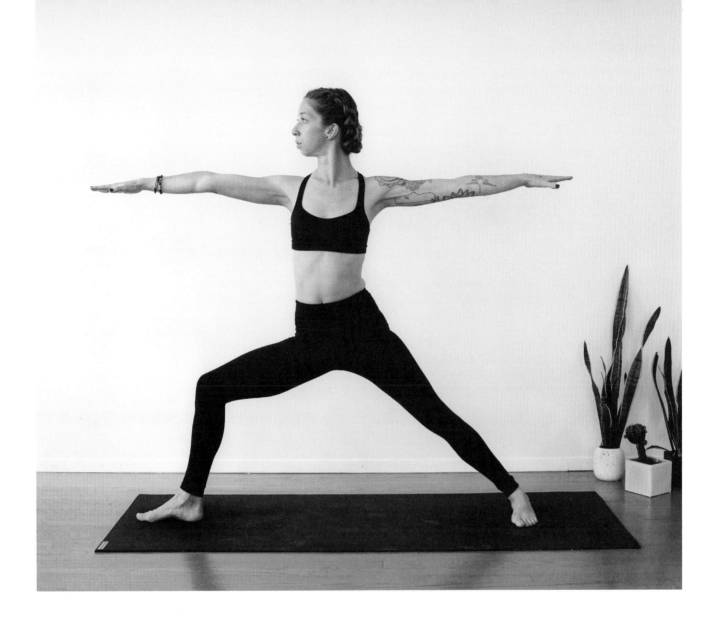

On an inhale exit the pose by bending your front knee and stepping your left leg lightly back into **WARRIOR TWO**.

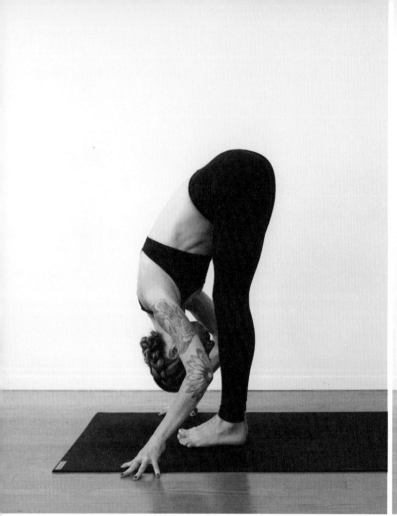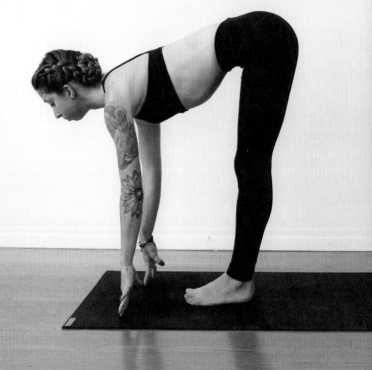

Cartwheel your hands down to the floor, framing your front foot. Step forward to **FORWARD FOLD**, with your feet together and your spine long.

Inhale, lifting your chest halfway up and bringing your hands to shins or thighs, into a **HALFWAY LIFT**.

Exhale, plant your palms, and step or hop back into
CHATURANGA DANDASANA.

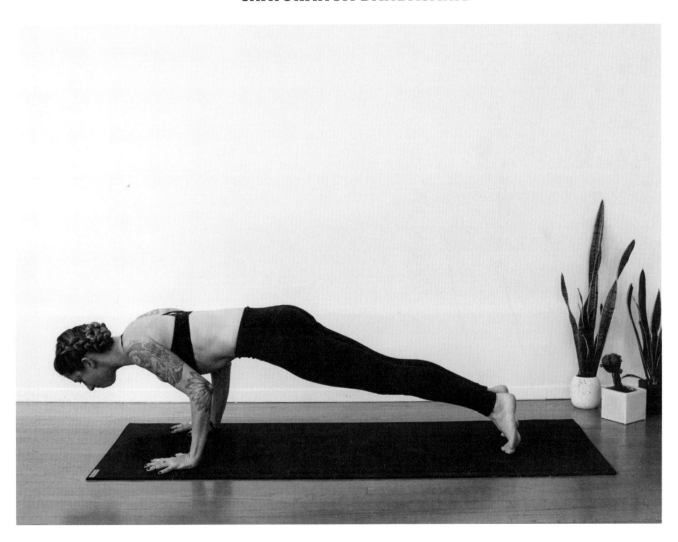

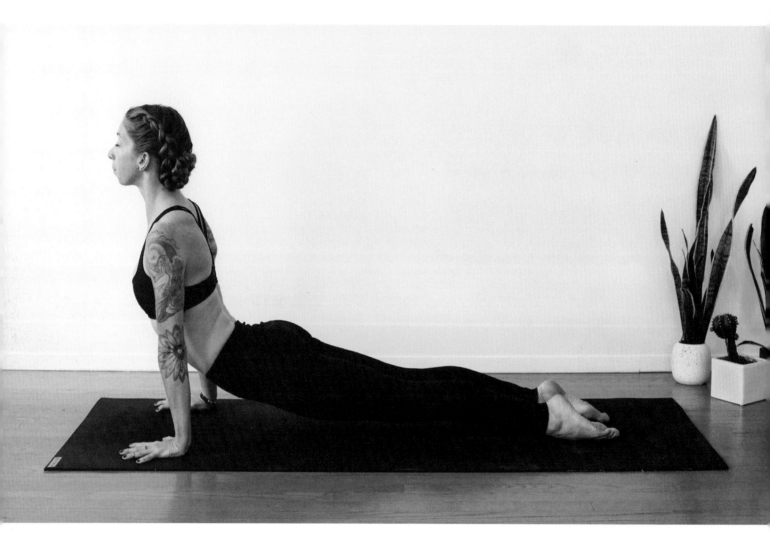

Move through your **VINYASA FLOW**
(**PLANK** to **UPWARD FACING DOG**), finishing in
DOWNWARD FACING DOG.

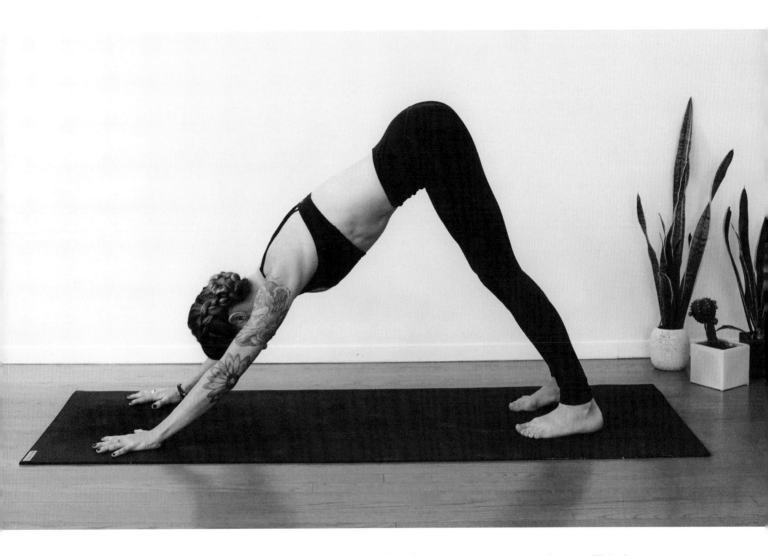

Rest before repeating the sequence on the left side. This flow can be practiced initially by holding the postures for around five breaths each, and then practiced again with one breath per movement for increased fluidity.

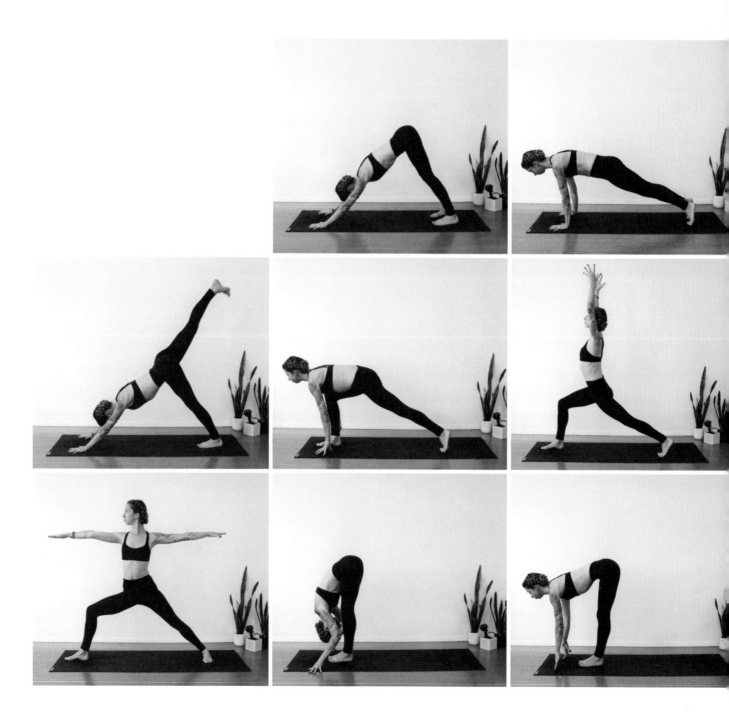

Quick Flow Guide: Y7 Flow

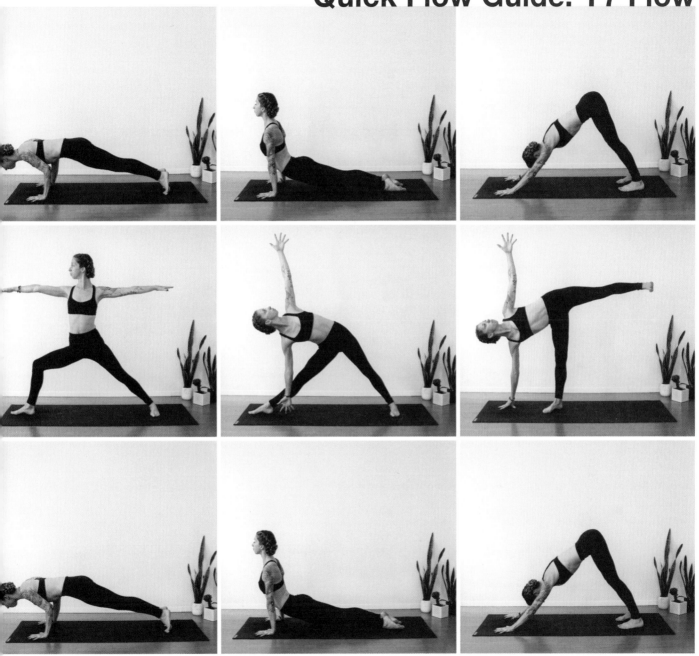

95

DIO

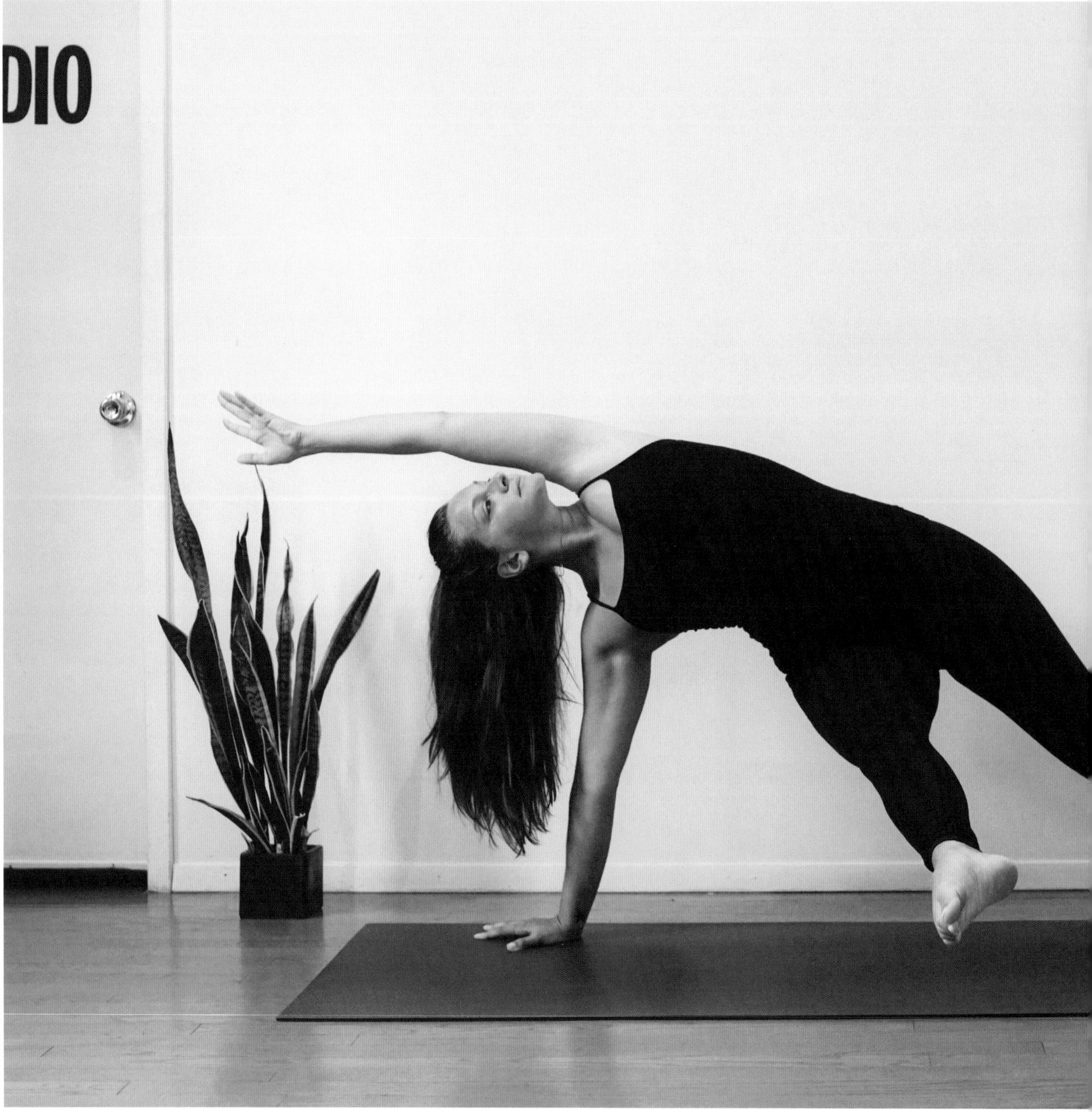

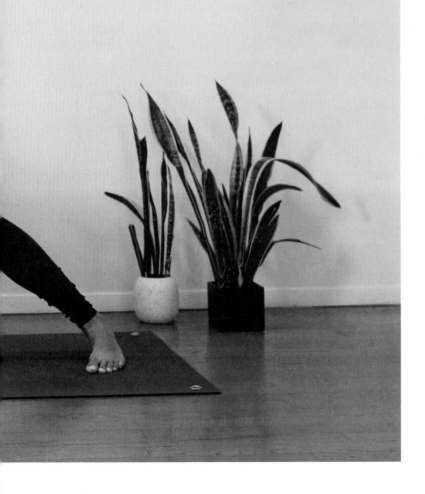

Y7 Mega Detox

(STEPH L.)

Steph is a 200-hour Registered Yoga Teacher (RYT), creator of the Y7 Mega Detox, and the director of teaching at Y7.

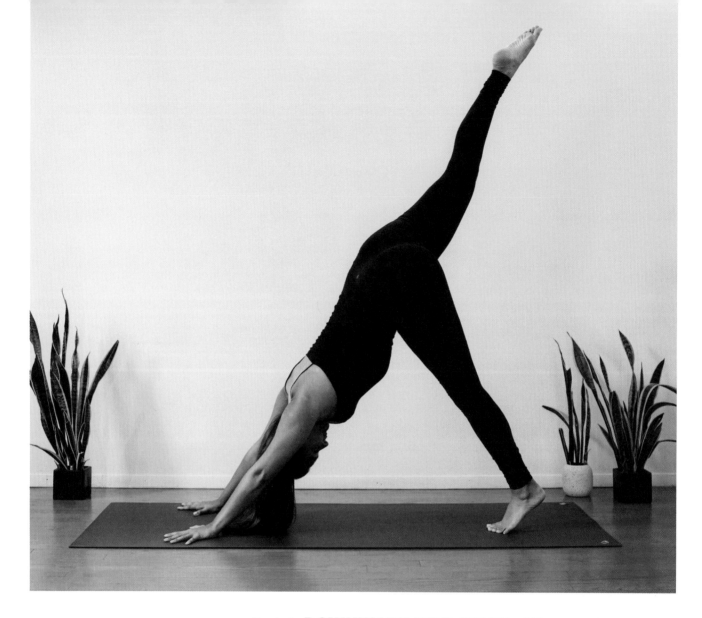

Begin in **DOWNWARD DOG SPLIT** by lifting your right leg high to the sky.

From this position, stack your right hip on top of the left hip, bending your right knee. Gently allow your right toes to meet the ground as you encourage your hips and heart to the sky, arriving in **ROCKSTAR POSE**.

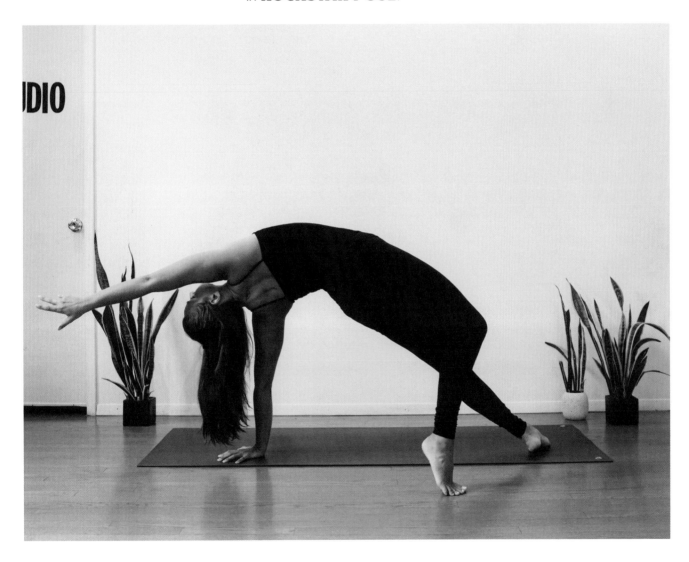

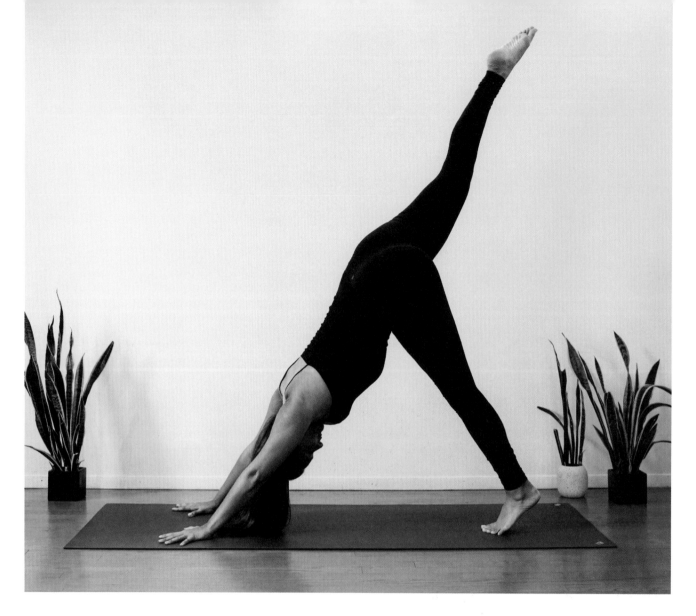

Unwind from Rockstar back into **DOWNWARD DOG SPLIT**.

From that position, draw your right knee to left elbow. Straighten the right leg out to the left as you spin your left heel down to the ground. Reach the left arm toward the sky and gaze up as you come into **FALLEN TRIANGLE**.

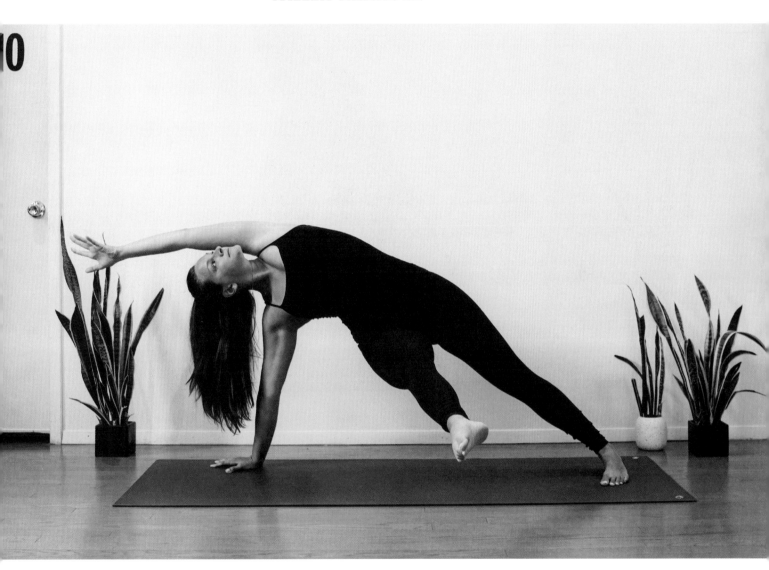

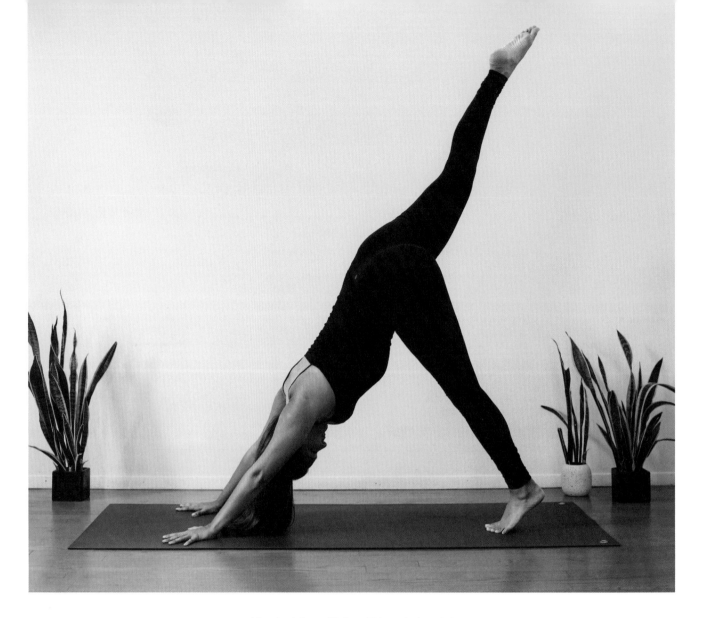

Unwind from Fallen Triangle back into
DOWNWARD DOG SPLIT.

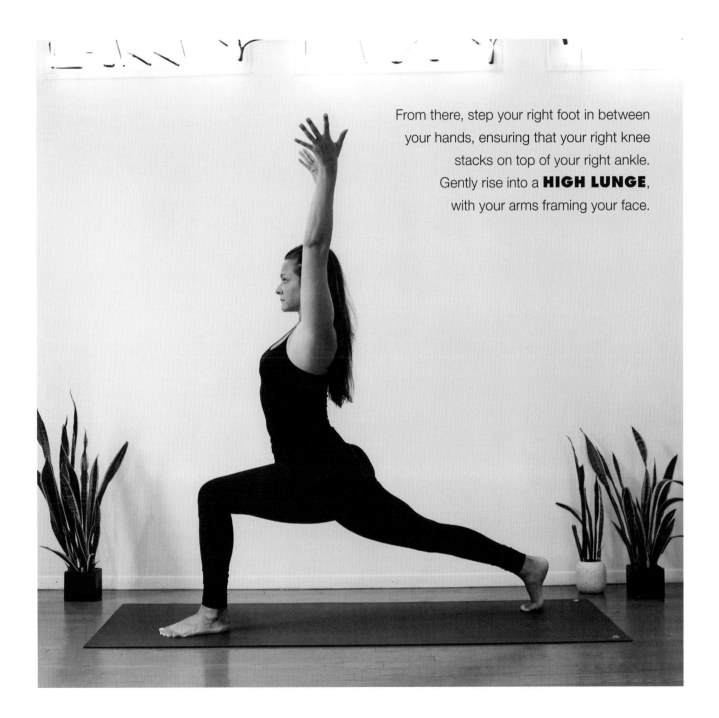

From there, step your right foot in between your hands, ensuring that your right knee stacks on top of your right ankle. Gently rise into a **HIGH LUNGE**, with your arms framing your face.

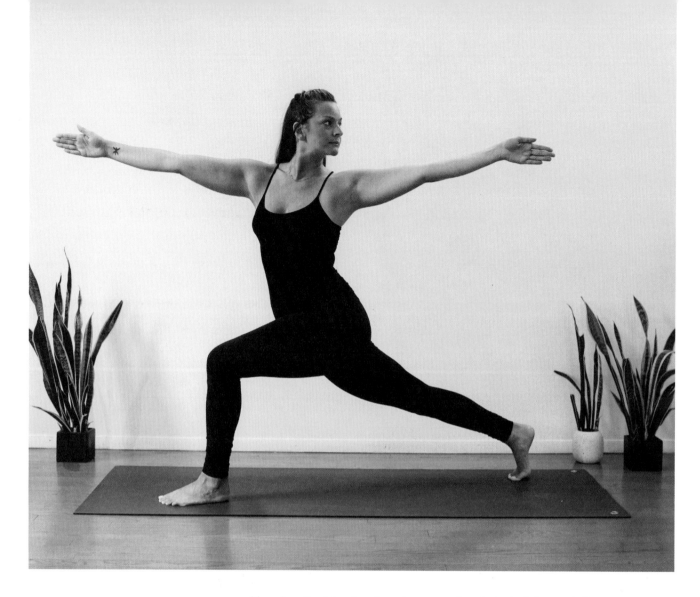

Keeping the hips level and square, begin to twist your left arm backward and right arm forward until you arrive in **HIGH LUNGE T-TWIST**, an upright twisting position. Continue to twist your chest and abdomen toward the left side as you work to keep your hips square to the front of your mat.

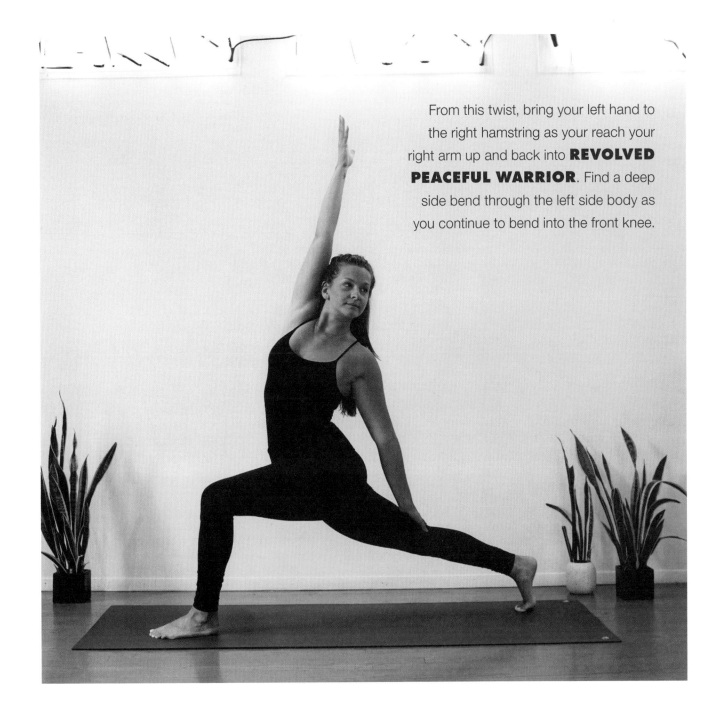

From this twist, bring your left hand to the right hamstring as your reach your right arm up and back into **REVOLVED PEACEFUL WARRIOR**. Find a deep side bend through the left side body as you continue to bend into the front knee.

Begin to draw your right elbow down and outside your left thigh. Your right palm will meet your left palm as you arrive in a **CLOSED PRAYER TWIST HIGH LUNGE**. Keep the back leg energized, and with each exhale deepen your twist as you gaze over your left shoulder.

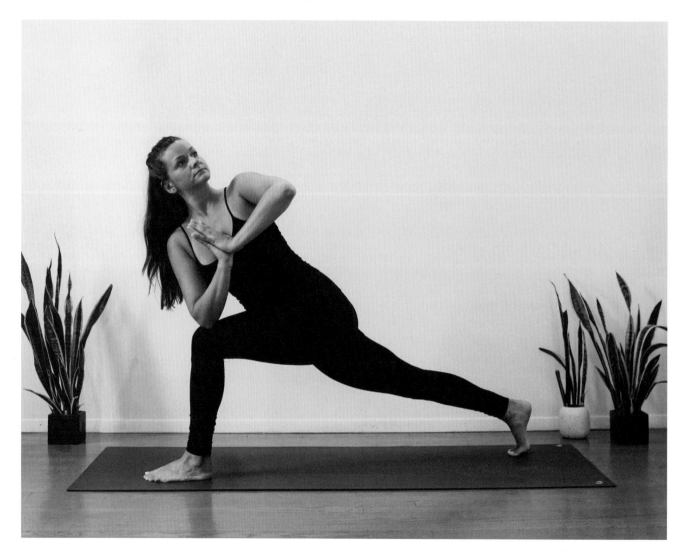

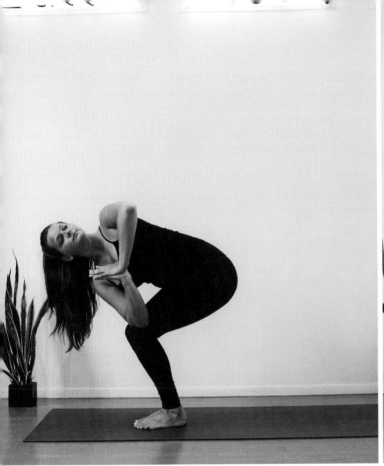

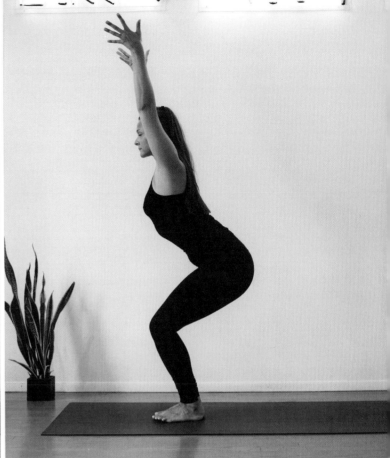

Shift your gaze toward the ground outside of your left foot. Shift your weight into your right foot as you gently step your right foot to meet your left foot, keeping the prayer twist at heart center. Ensure your knees are aligned with one another and sit your weight back into your heels as you settle into your **CHAIR TWIST**. Keep your hips level, and with each exhale encourage a deeper twist as you gaze over your left shoulder.

Gently unwind out of your twist, into **CHAIR**, until your torso faces forward and your arms frame your face. Sit your weight into your heels and stack your knees over your ankles.

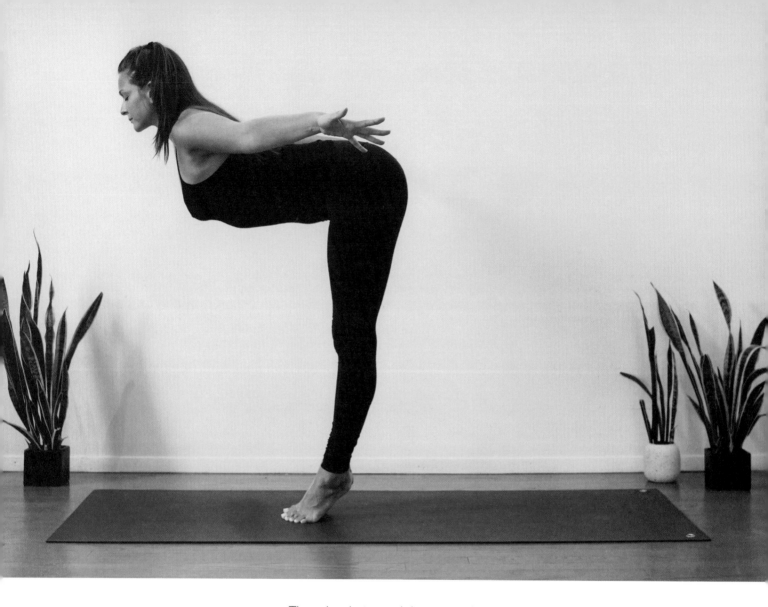

Then, begin to straighten your legs and wind your arms behind you. Come high onto your tiptoes into **DIVERS**—encourage your heels together and your weight into your big toes. Feel your tailbone draw to the back of your mat as your heart draws to the front of the mat. Engage the abdomen to create stability.

From Divers, gently bend your knees out to the sides, creating a diamond shape with your legs. Lean your upper body down and plant your palms under your shoulders, spreading wide through the fingers. Keep your tail up high as you wedge your knees directly into your armpits. Shift your gaze and heart forward as you float one foot off the ground, and then the other foot. Suck the navel up to find your engagement in the core as you grip the ground with your fingertips, coming into **CROW POSE**.

Repeat the full sequence on your other side.

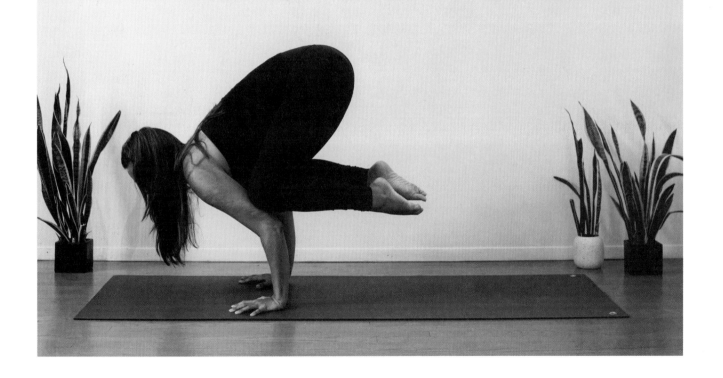

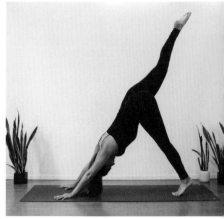

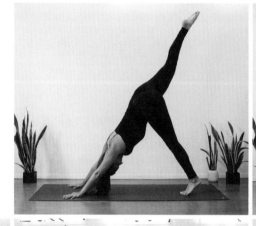

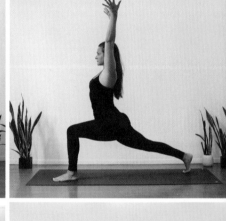

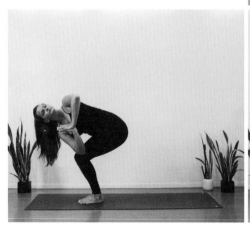

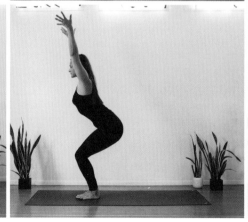

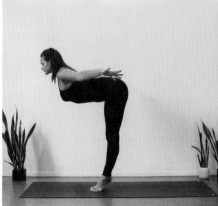

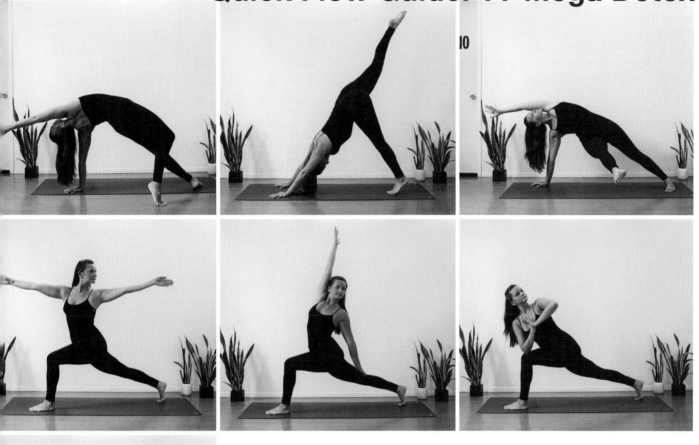

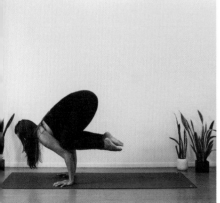

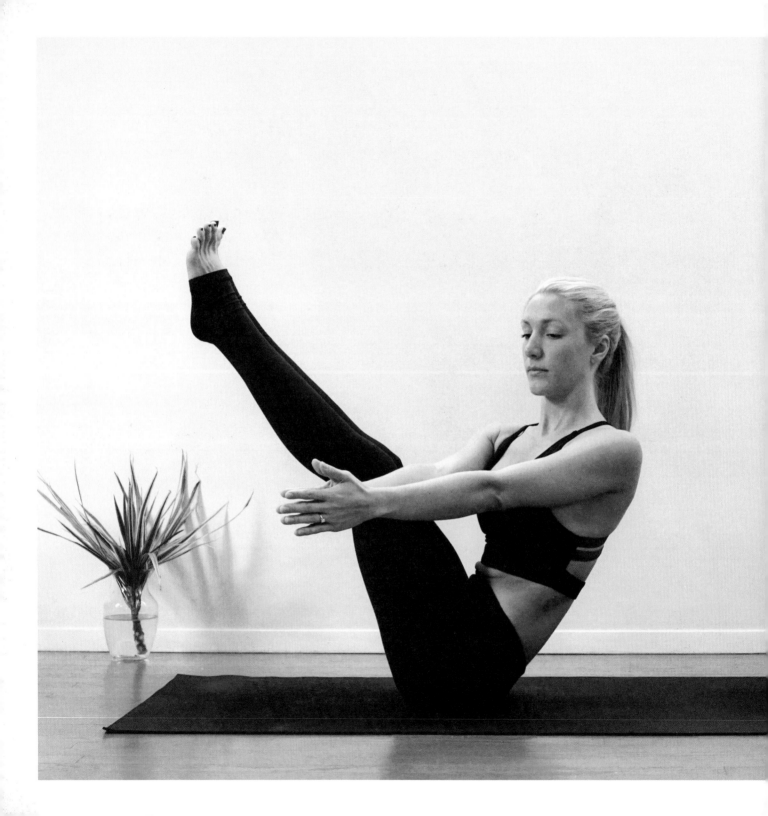

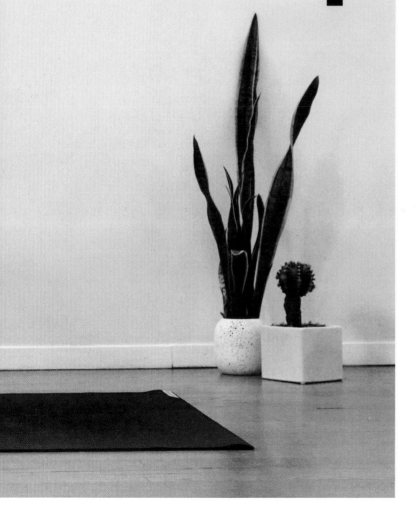

Abs&Ass Sequence

(KRISTIN L.)

Kristin is a 200-hour Experienced Registered Yoga Teacher (ERYT)/ Registered Prenatal Yoga Teacher (RPYT) and a Teaching Manager at Y7 Studio.

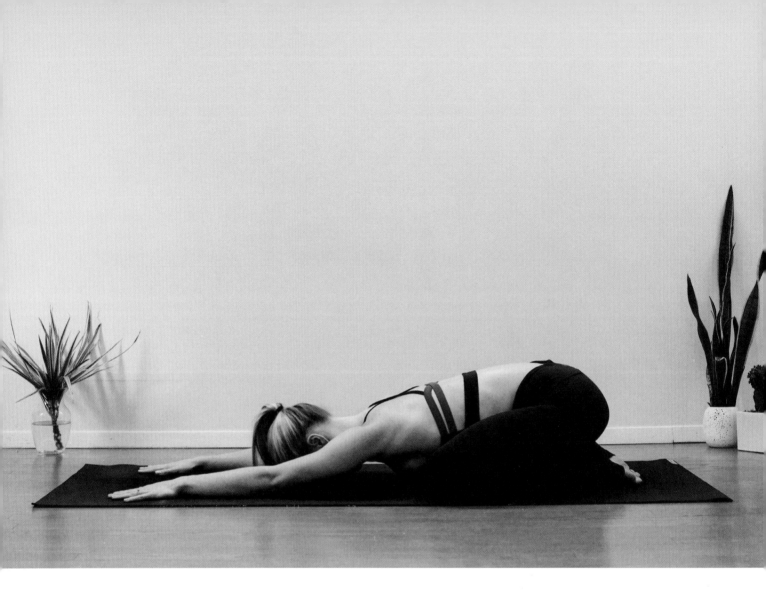

Start in **CHILD'S POSE** with your knees out wide and your big toes together. Allow your forehead to rest comfortably on the mat as you sink your hips back toward your heels.

Come up onto hands and knees, to **TABLETOP**.
Make sure your wrists are under your shoulders, and your
knees under your hips. Draw your navel to your spine to
engage the core and create a flat back.

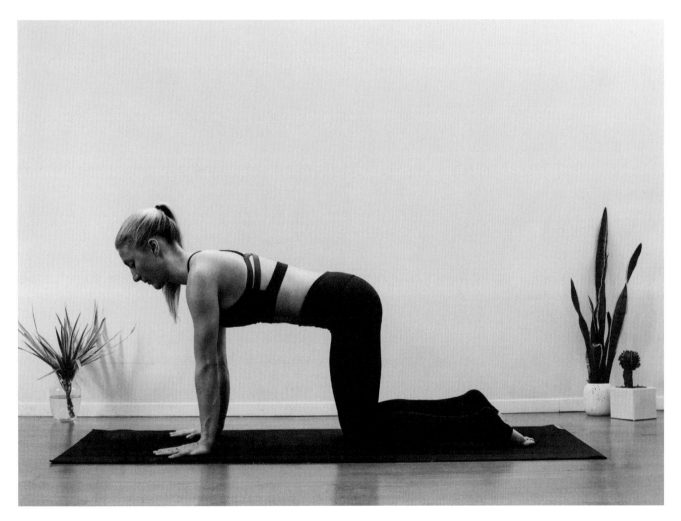

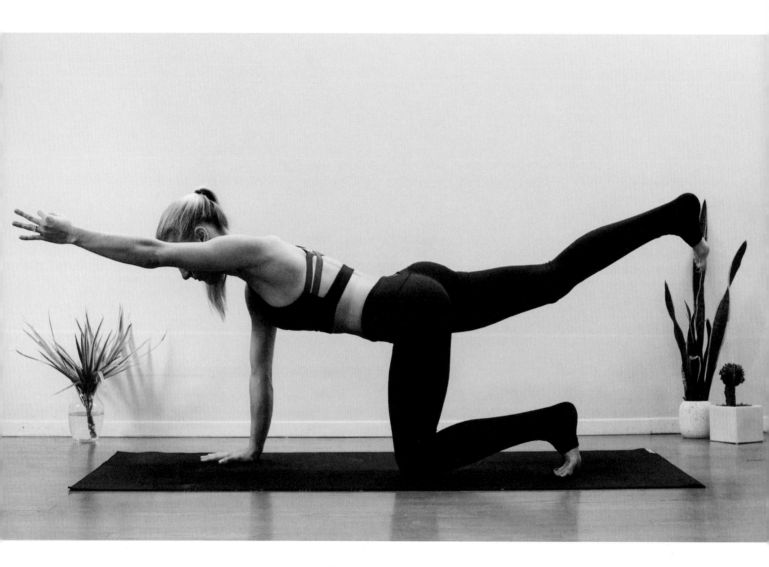

From Tabletop, extend your right leg back as you reach your left arm forward, coming into a **BALANCING TABLETOP** position. Continue to draw the belly in.

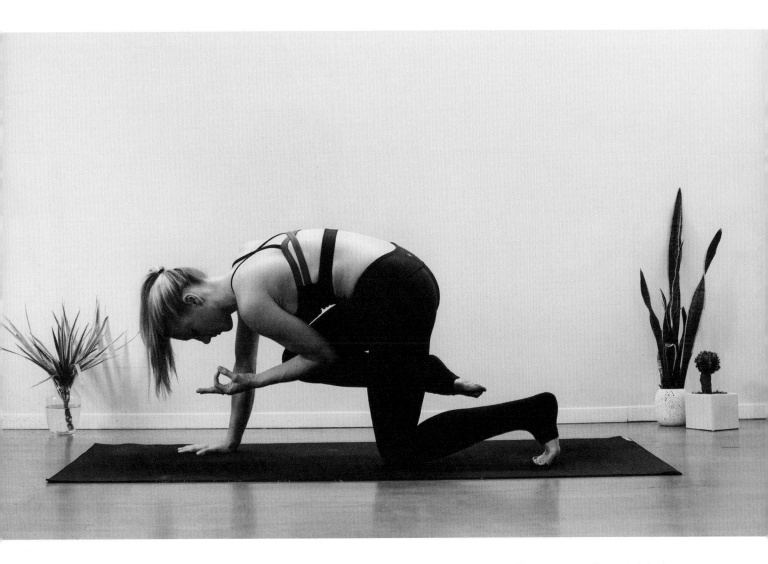

Now you'll use balancing tabletop to work your core. As you inhale, reach your arm and leg away from one another, as you exhale curl and round your back to the ceiling as you draw your elbow to your knee. Repeat this three to five times.

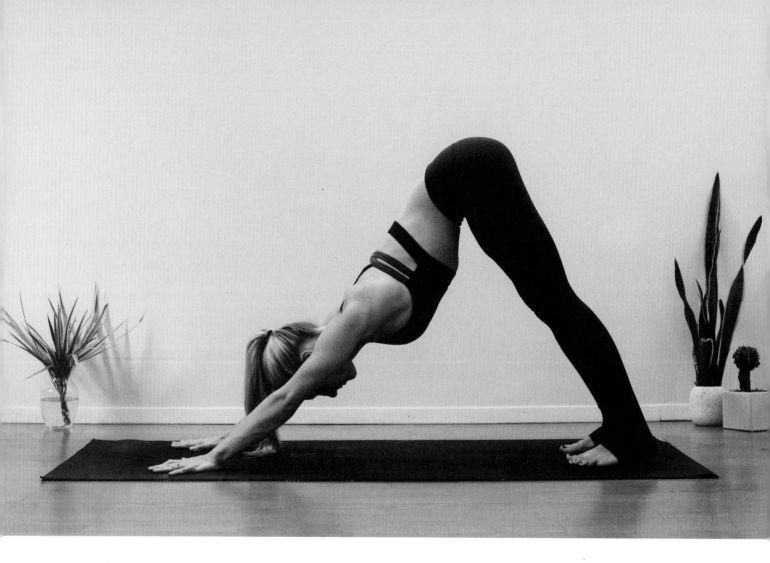

From Tabletop tuck your toes, lift your hips, and make your way into a **DOWNWARD FACING DOG**. Double-check that your fingers are spread wide, with your peace fingers—index and middle fingers—pointing forward, and ground down through all the knuckles in your hands to take the weight from your wrists into your fingertips. Lift your hips up high to the ceiling as you press your thighbones back and sink your heels to the ground.

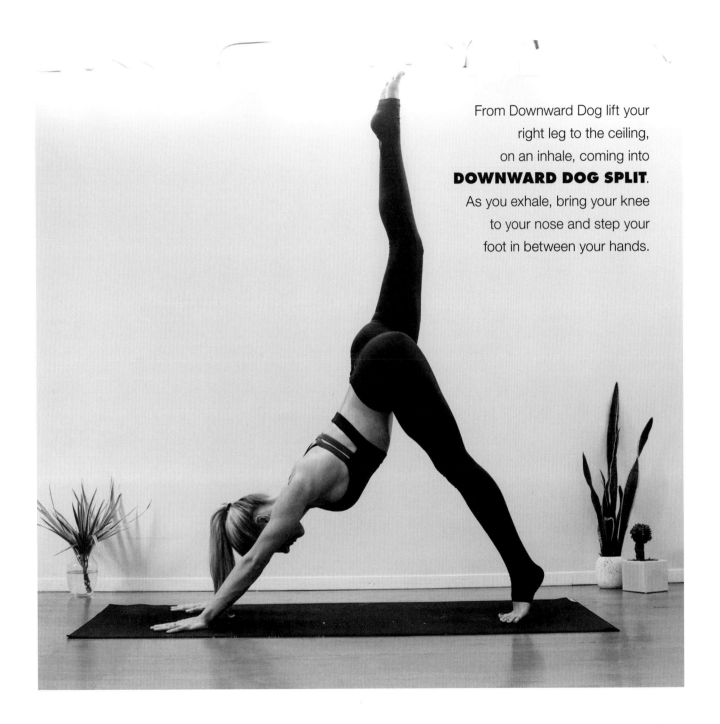

From Downward Dog lift your right leg to the ceiling, on an inhale, coming into **DOWNWARD DOG SPLIT**. As you exhale, bring your knee to your nose and step your foot in between your hands.

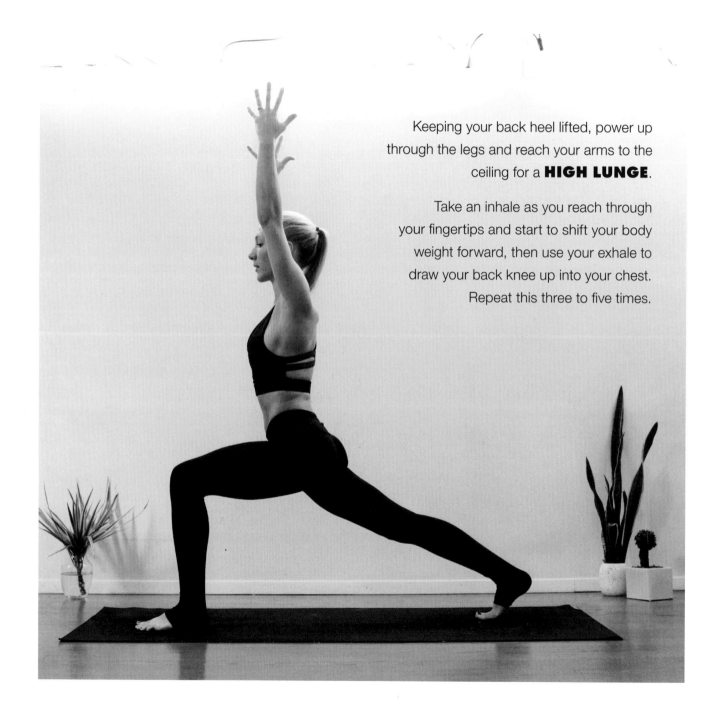

Keeping your back heel lifted, power up through the legs and reach your arms to the ceiling for a **HIGH LUNGE**.

Take an inhale as you reach through your fingertips and start to shift your body weight forward, then use your exhale to draw your back knee up into your chest. Repeat this three to five times.

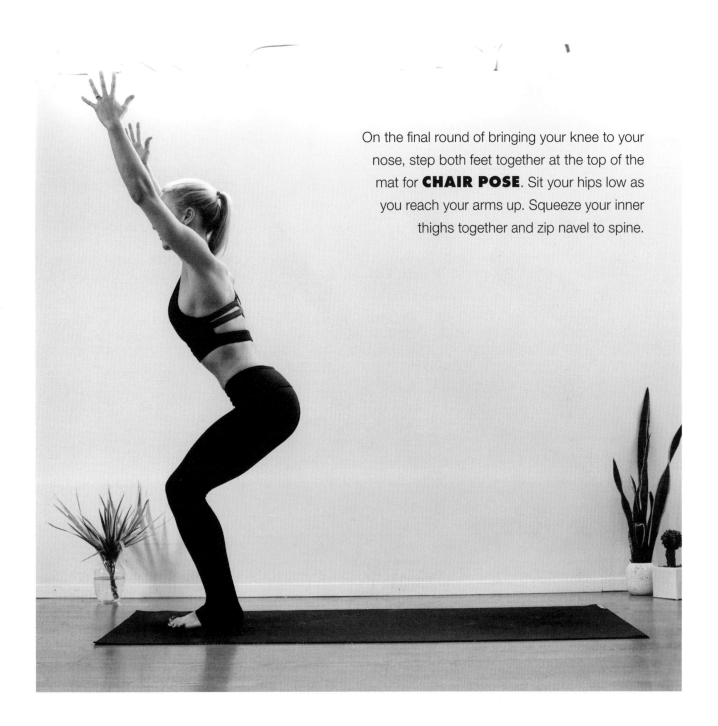

On the final round of bringing your knee to your nose, step both feet together at the top of the mat for **CHAIR POSE**. Sit your hips low as you reach your arms up. Squeeze your inner thighs together and zip navel to spine.

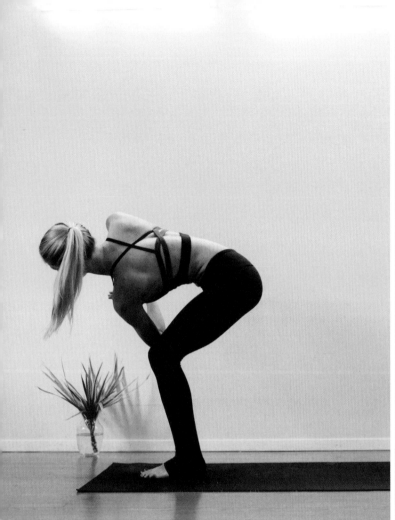
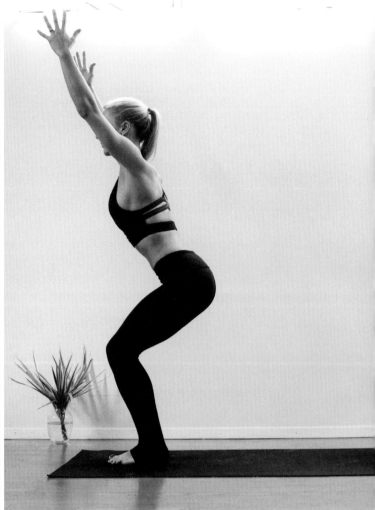

From Chair, bring your hands to heart center in prayer position. As you inhale, lift your chest toward your thumbs and roll your shoulder blades down your back, as you exhale twist to the right, hooking your left elbow outside of your right knee as you come into **TWISTED CHAIR**. Hold for three to five breaths.

On an inhale return to **CHAIR POSE**.

With your arms reaching up, and as you exhale, sit all the way down onto your sit bones for **BOAT POSE**. For a modified variation, bring your hands to your hamstrings. Bring your shins parallel to the floor, squeeze your inner thighs together, draw your belly up and in, and lift the center of the chest to the ceiling while keeping the shoulders relaxed.

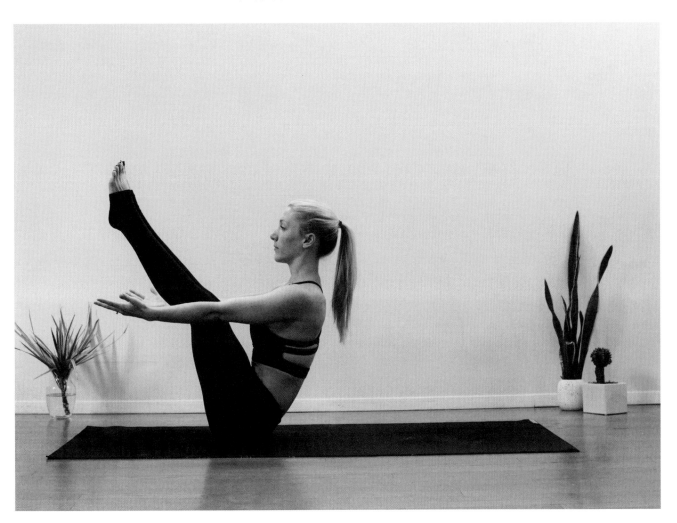

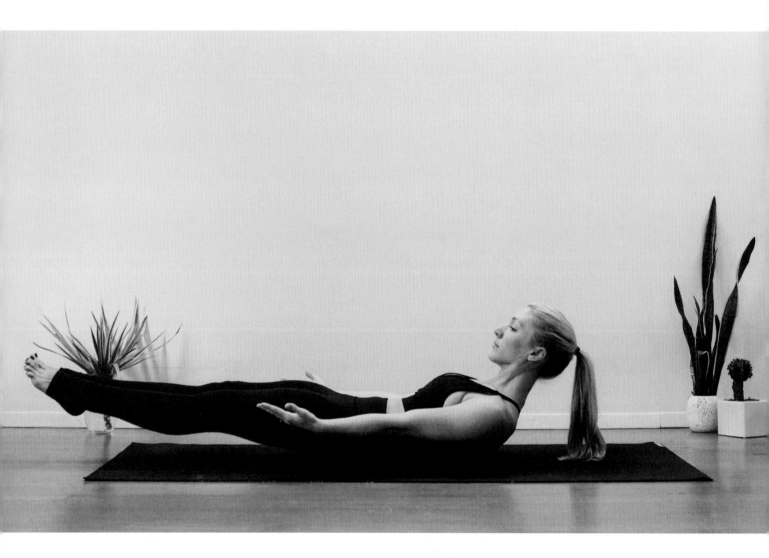

As you inhale lower into **LOW BOAT POSE**—your lower back will be on the mat with everything else hovering. Keep your belly drawing in.

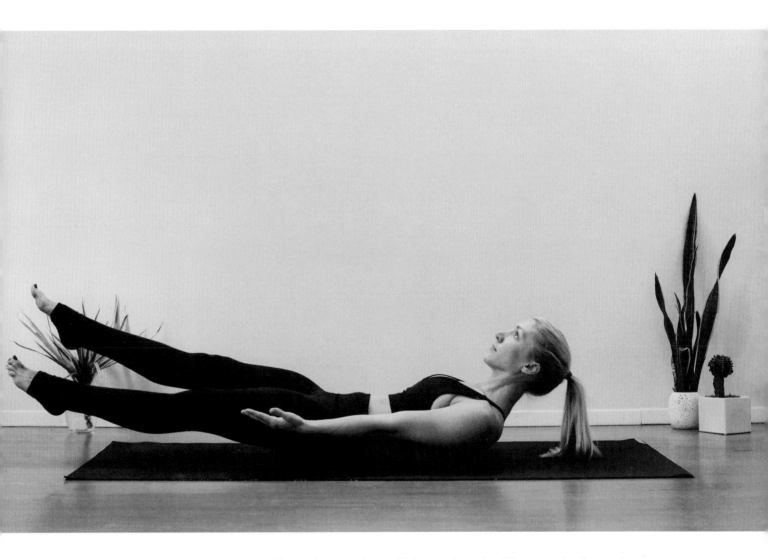

From there, scissor-kick your legs for 30 seconds, then release onto your back and hug your knees to your chest.

Repeat the full sequence on your left side.

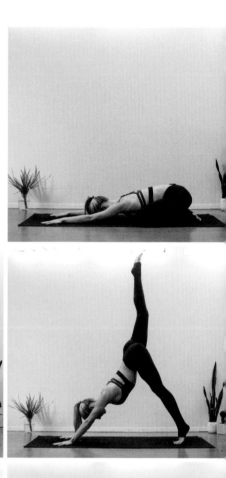

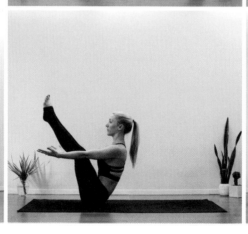

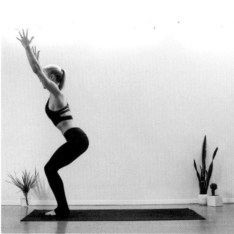

Quick Flow Guide: Abs & Ass Sequence

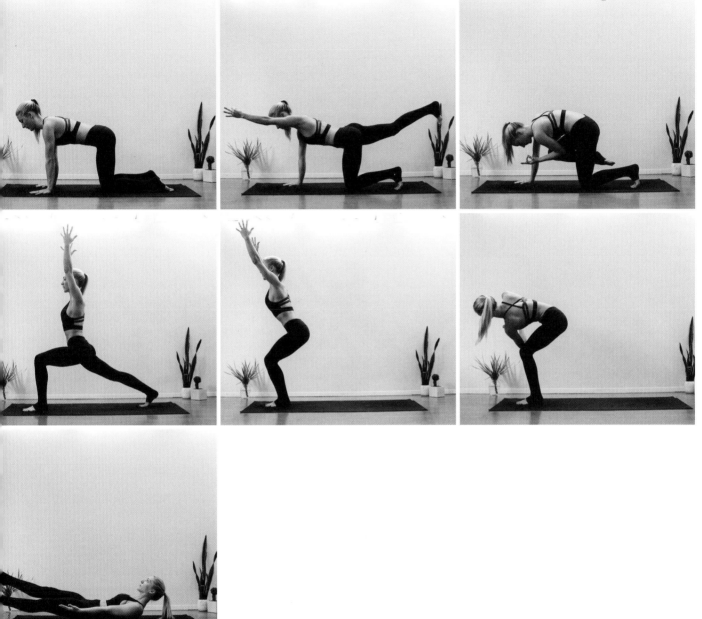

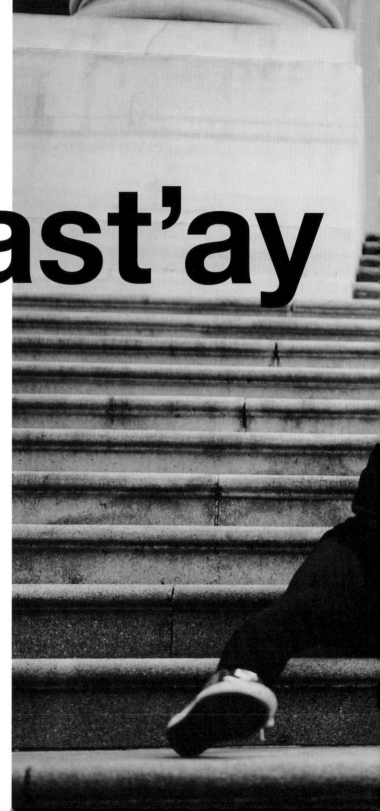

PART 3

Namast'ay Fly

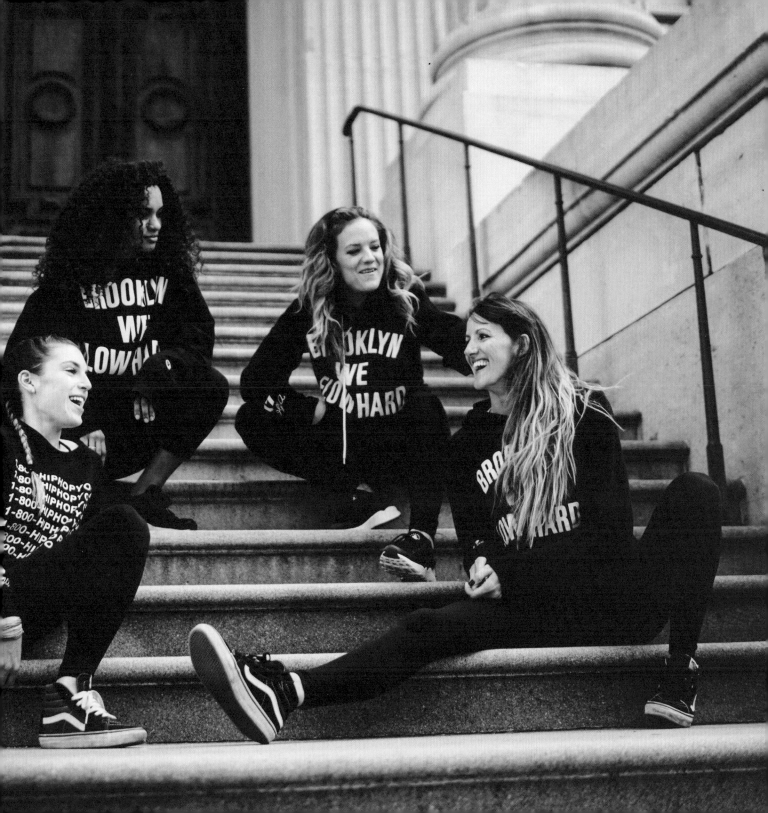

FINDING BALANCE

We Flow Hard—that's our motto at Y7, and we bring that energy to everything we do. Pushing yourself to grow—in your practice and your life—is a major part of our philosophy. You've got to hustle, but that doesn't mean you need to go at 110 percent all the time. In fact, if yoga teaches us anything, it's that finding balance is the key to real growth—that harmony between the body and the mind, movement and breath, on the mat isn't just for your workout.

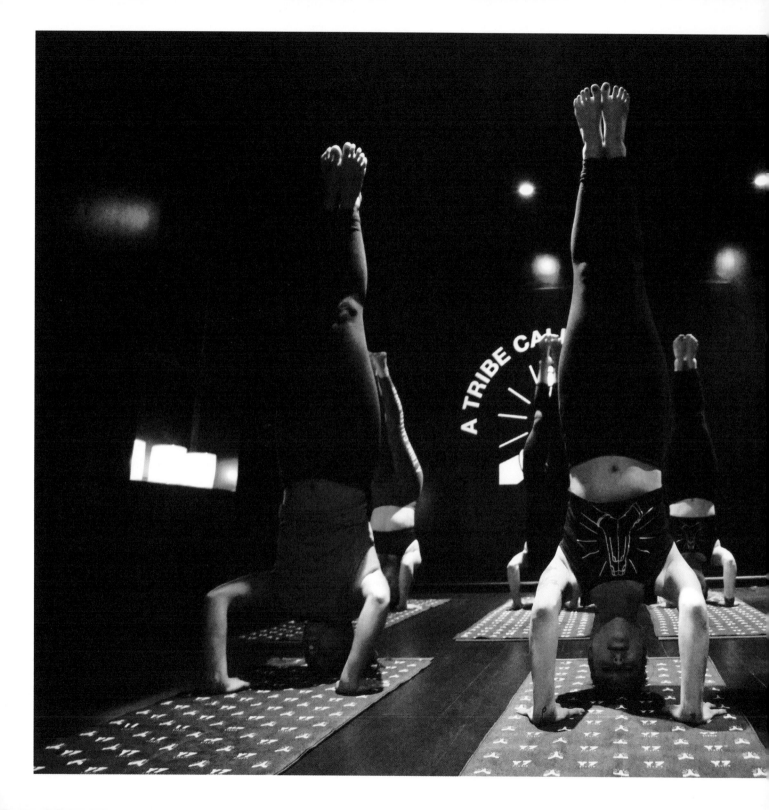

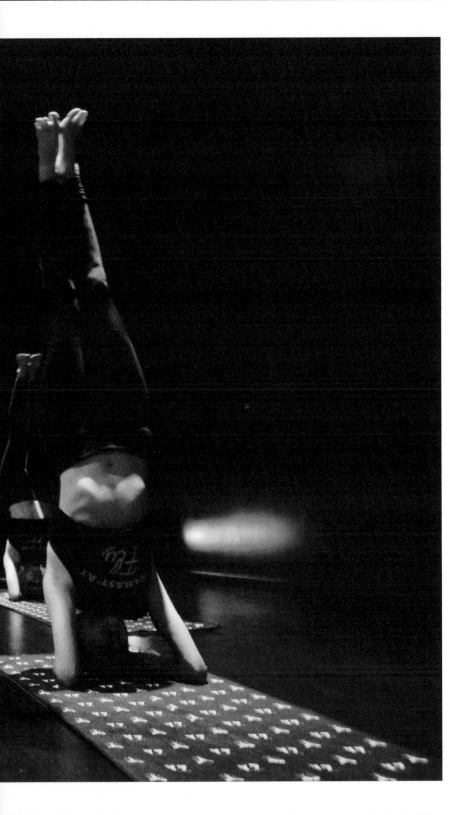

But we get a lot of messages from the world about what a balanced, "yogi" lifestyle is all about. We see images of pious meditating vegans looking serene as they spend hours a day on the mat. And that's just not most of us. Don't get me wrong: I love a meditating vegan. But I'm not one. And you don't have to be one either to feel the benefits of a yoga practice and a yogi lifestyle every day.

The key for me, and for the tribe we've created at Y7, is to figure out what aspects of the practice fit into our real life. Come to the mat when you can, meditate when you can, eat food that nourishes your body without depriving yourself. And know that depriving yourself of the things you love—whether that's a cocktail, a night out dancing, or a week off from your yoga practice—isn't going to make your practice better.

These are the tips and ideas that help me create a life that feels balanced—one where I see the people I love, feel satisfied with my choices, and *get shit done*. Take the ones that serve you and leave the rest; that's the philosophy that the best yogis I know follow.

WORKING ON YOUR PRACTICE

Taking your first class and beginning your journey with yoga can be daunting. You walk into the studio and start hearing unfamiliar Sanskrit words; you're told to get into physical poses you didn't know your body could possibly go into; and on top of that sutras (rules or teachings), mantras (sounds and chants), and pranayamas (breathing patterns) all get brought in. As a new student, how do you navigate through all that information? And even for those who are not new to the practice, how do you balance all of the different components of yoga?

One of the most important things to know when you begin a yoga practice is that every person's body is different. This might sound like a basic concept, but it is something I struggled with for a long time—and I'm not the only one. I thought that I had to look exactly like a yoga model, or be perfect in my postures, to get the benefits of the practice. But what I've learned over time is that this is *not* true at all. It's a harmful belief, and it isn't what yoga is truly about. Your body is unlike anyone else's, and that is a beautiful thing. You may never be able to do a Forearm Stand, you may never even be able to touch your toes, and that is *okay*. As long as you are engaging the muscles that are central to the asana (pose) and your alignment is correct, you are reaping the physical benefits of the pose.

It is called a yoga *practice* for a reason. If there's only one thing you take away from this book, it's that. We are all *practicing*, no one is perfect, everyone is working to be better. It can be really easy to focus on setting a goal when it comes to yoga, especially when you're beginning your practice (e.g., I am going to do yoga because I want to nail a handstand). That's a very admirable goal, and I don't want to discourage anyone from

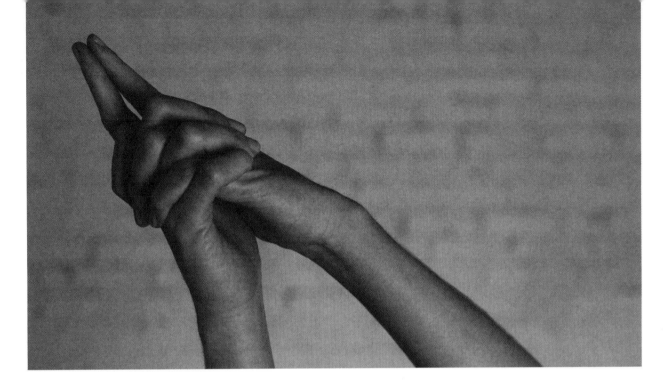

pushing themself to deepen their practice. But achieving a specific goal is not the *point* of the practice.

What we want to encourage at Y7 is the ability to sit with yourself during uncomfortable moments—something that is valuable on the mat and off. In a challenging pose we want you to be able to breathe through the shaking muscles, concentrating on the feeling and not the fear. That is the real skill, and it teaches you the ability to be in the present moment. Bringing awareness to these elements of yoga—the breath, the connection of mind and body, the sensation of exploring your limits—will help you in other areas of your life as well. The techniques you practice on the mat, regardless of your technical ability, can benefit you in so many ways from being more focused on current relationships to not being afraid of the outcome of a certain action. By taking this approach to yoga, you will learn to live in a more authentic way, seeing what will happen if you take a chance rather than being afraid. And, if you ask me, that's a much better accomplishment than doing a Handstand.

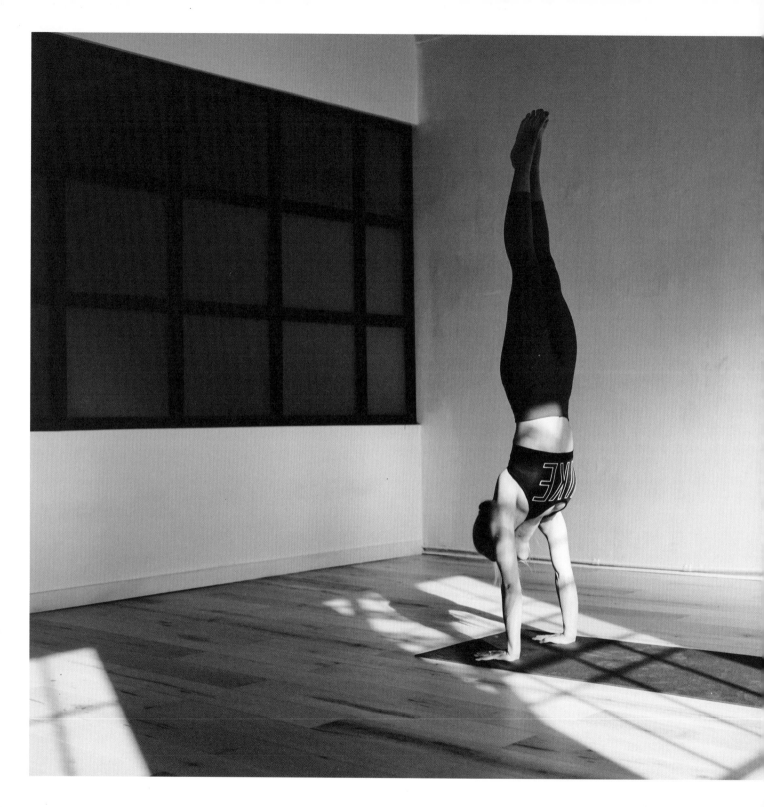

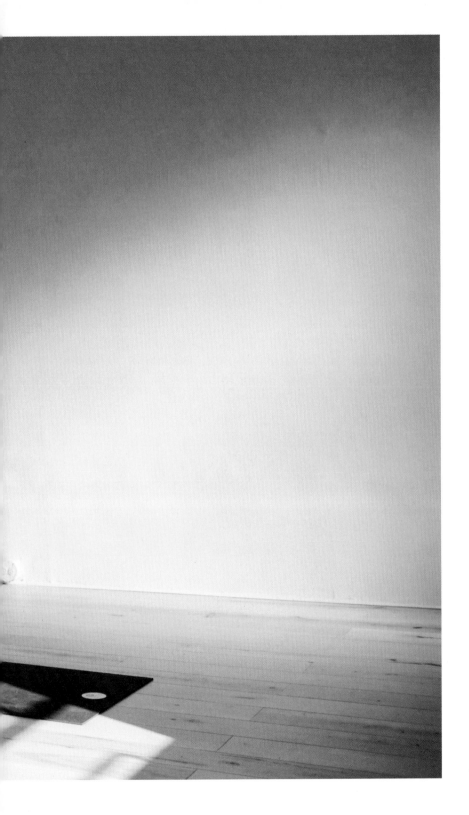

LOVING YOURSELF

Yoga is about you—*your* body, *your* mind. That's an amazing, powerful concept, but it isn't always the easiest ideal to live up to. We are typically our own harshest critics, constantly comparing ourselves to others or an idealized version of how we should be. How awful is that!?

Those negative vibes don't need to be a part of your life, and they definitely don't need to be a part of your yoga practice. At Y7 we aim to eliminate that self-doubt, instead creating a feeling of love and gratitude for everything that we are able to bring to the table. In the studio we've worked to cultivate that positive energy by taking out mirrors and lighting the space exclusively with candles, setting up an environment that is safe. No one can see you if you fall, so you might as well try!

The bottom line is that you need to be able to sit with yourself. This core principle lies at the heart of yoga, and it's not a coincidence that it's also a key part of loving yourself as you are. At the end of the day, if you eliminate all the competition and pressure you feel from the outside world, you are just left with yourself. You are the only person you answer to. No one else can tell you if you tried your best or if you gave it your all—knowing the answers to those questions has to come from within.

It can be really hard to stop all of the outside noise from getting in the way of your inner peace. And that's where yoga comes in. A yoga practice is a work-out for the mind. It challenges you to ignore the little voice in your head—the one that tells you your body is tired or you just can't do it. The secret that yoga teaches is that you *can*. You truly can do what you put your mind to.

You'll find that the confidence you cultivate inside the studio and in your home practice will begin to present itself in other areas of your life. Trust me, I'm not saying that this is easy. I am not even close to being at complete peace with myself. I constantly find my mind wandering, and I still compare myself to others who seem to have it all figured out. But I try to use the peace I've developed through yoga to come back to who I am, the things that give me joy, and the things that inspire me to be better. And I remember those little moments of struggle that I have overcome—the days when I held Chair Pose for a little longer than I thought I could, the knowledge that I pushed myself even though I was tired. It's those everyday victories that we need to celebrate and that bring us closer to the self-love and acceptance that yoga teaches. Loving yourself comes from so much more than outside validation. It comes from knowing that where you are today is good enough. And if you are not happy with that, understand that tomorrow is a new day and a chance for growth.

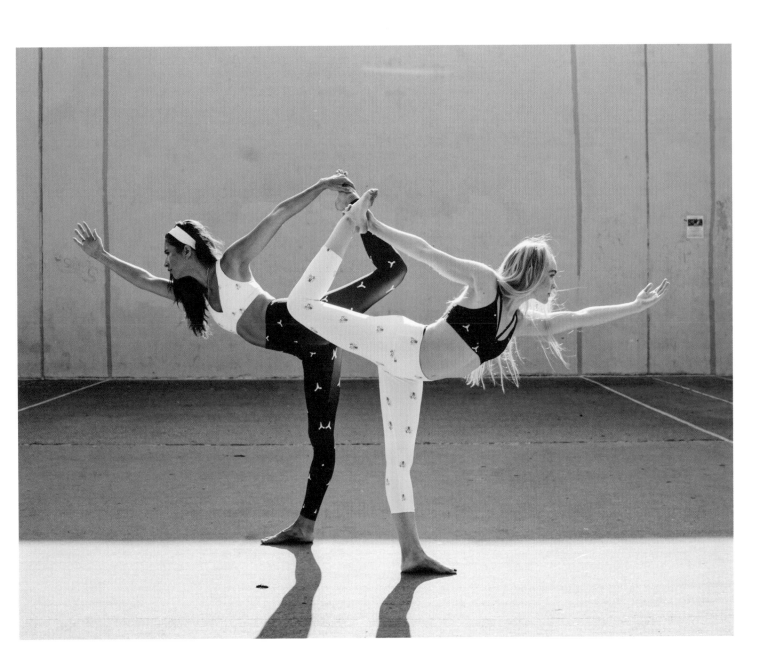

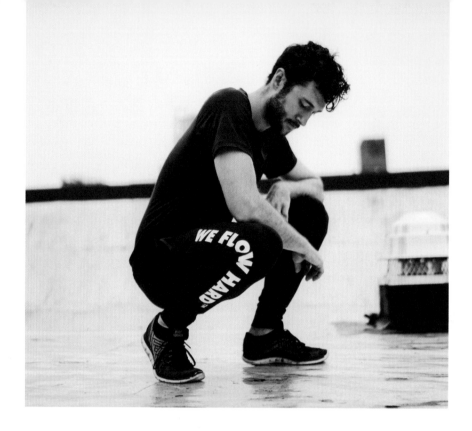

UNPLUGGING

Let's face it: we live in a fast-paced world. There are so many distractions in our lives that hinder our ability to unplug. There is always something that we need to do, always somewhere to be, always something to check off our to-do lists. How do we set aside all of those thoughts for even five minutes, let alone for an entire hourlong yoga class?! Just writing this makes it seem nearly impossible.

As tempting as it is to stay constantly plugged in, checking item after item off of those endless to-do lists, no one can run on empty. How can we do all of the things we need to in life—from your exciting side hustle to mundane grocery shopping—but still be personally charged up? The answer is simple:

you need to take time for yourself. I know, I know—easier said than done! But yoga teaches us many techniques to help us with this challenging task. One of the best lessons we can learn from yoga is that it's the quality of the recharging that matters, not the time it takes. You do not need to meditate for three hours a day to unplug. You need to find something that works for you.

When I am feeling stressed or overwhelmed with work or projects, I remind myself that I'm not going to be able to do my best unless I am in a good place. I step back. I take ten minutes to walk away from what I am doing. I love doing a small meditation during this time, either on my own (see page 171) or with a guided app like Headspace. I'll do a breathing exercise and focus on the inhales and exhales, bringing myself back to the present moment. I ask myself some centering questions: what is important now, in this moment? By taking a small break from distractions, technology, and other people, I bring myself back to the task at hand, instead of focusing on what *could* happen if I don't do something, or what *might* happen if someone doesn't do what I ask. Yoga is ultimately an individual practice, and it teaches us that we can only control our own actions—what others do is outside of our control.

The practice also teaches the importance of setting boundaries for yourself. Carving out a space without technology is difficult, but it's a crucial way to bring the lessons from yoga into your everyday life—and it makes such a difference. If you find that you get into bed at 10:00 p.m., but are up for two hours on your phone looking at Snapchat, that's not creating healthy boundaries for yourself. We've all been there: waking up tired in the morning and wondering where the time went. Consider plugging your phone in on the other side of the room. Force yourself to just be in bed. That's it. The discipline that you cultivate on the mat—that force inside that allows you to hold your poses even when you want to give up—isn't just about your workout. Unplugging from distraction can be tough, but taking time for yourself and finding something that brings you joy will ultimately make you a more productive and happy person.

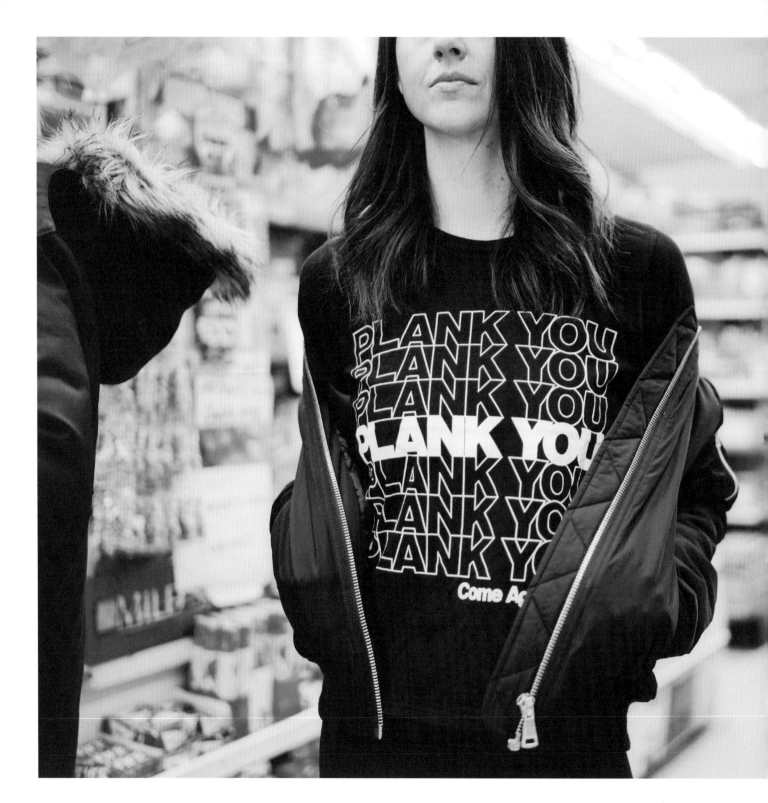

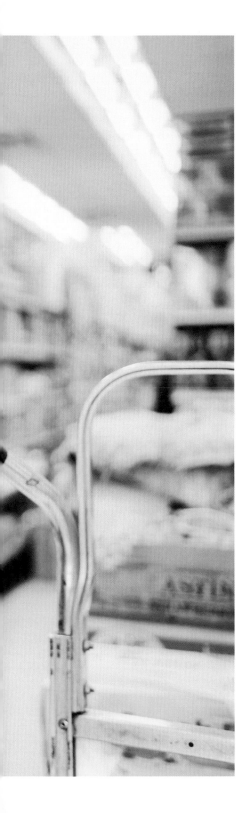

NOURISHING YOUR BODY

A theme that we constantly come back to at Y7 is that everyone is different. This is true for how our bodies move, and it's just as true when it comes to how to care for them. I know that in order for me to be at my best I need at least six to eight hours of solid sleep—but I also know other people who can be good on five. The same goes for food and workouts. In order for us to care for and honor ourselves, we must recognize what we need in order to be at our best. Of course we are all going to slip up. (I am guilty of drinking half my weight in wine and staying out until 4:00 a.m.—no one is perfect.)

Ultimately, to care for yourself means to be kind to yourself. We need to eat good food, drink good drinks, and be with the people who inspire and love us.

ACHIEVING BALANCED NUTRITION

Balance—it is a major key to happiness and overall well-being. And it seems like a relatively simple concept. However, as we all know, things that seem basic are often easier said than done. For me, achieving balanced nutrition has been about finding out what works for my body. Every body is unique. This is true when it comes to your yoga practice, and it is just as true when it comes to nutrition.

The concept of bio-individuality is a great benchmark to figure out what works for you and your body. Here's a personal example: No-carb diets do not work for me. They just don't. I don't lose fat, and I actually feel more sluggish and low energy. I am not a scientist, so I won't try to speculate on why this is—and it most certainly does not mean that I should eat pizza for three meals a day (even though I would). The point of this story is that I found that I am my healthiest and happiest when I have grains and carbohydrates in my diet. It took *years* for me to figure this out, and until I did, I was a huge fad dieter. During that time, I tried every new theory that came out. I tried a juice cleanse (I fainted on the subway platform my second morning in). I tried going vegan (I gained ten pounds and my skin broke out). I tried eliminating carbs (I had zero energy and was very irritable). None of these quick fixes gave me the results I wanted—and they all threw my body out of balance.

Things finally changed for me when I really started to listen to my body, understanding its rhythms and the things that fueled it best. This process of self-discovery also led to a passionate interest in nutrition—so much so that I studied to become a certified Health Coach through the Institute for Integrative Nutrition. Learning about the way nutrition could impact the

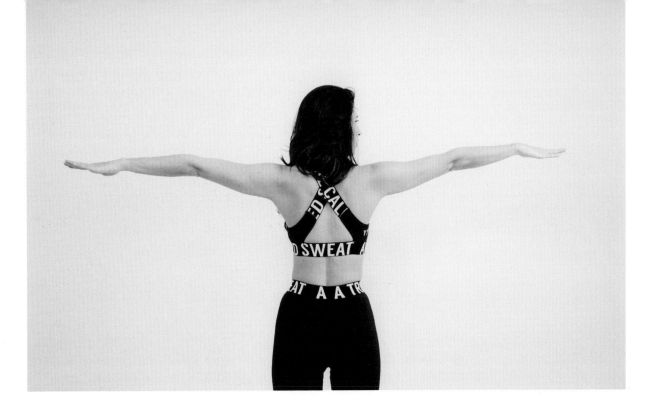

body made so many things clear to me, and I really started to pay attention to what I was putting in my body and how it reacted afterward.

There isn't just one way to approach nutrition, and it can sometimes feel overwhelming to start thinking about it in a more cohesive way. For me, it was important to know what my baseline was—to know how my body reacted to different foods.

To get myself on the right track, I did my own detox (I use the word "detox" loosely here—a balanced approach to nutrition isn't about deprivation, but about knowing what your body does and doesn't like). For three days I eliminated all dairy, sugar, and carbohydrates. My diet was focused around green vegetables and proteins—this meant hard-boiled eggs for breakfast, a green salad for lunch (dressed with lemon juice), and grilled salmon with steamed green vegetables for dinner. On the fourth day I added back in

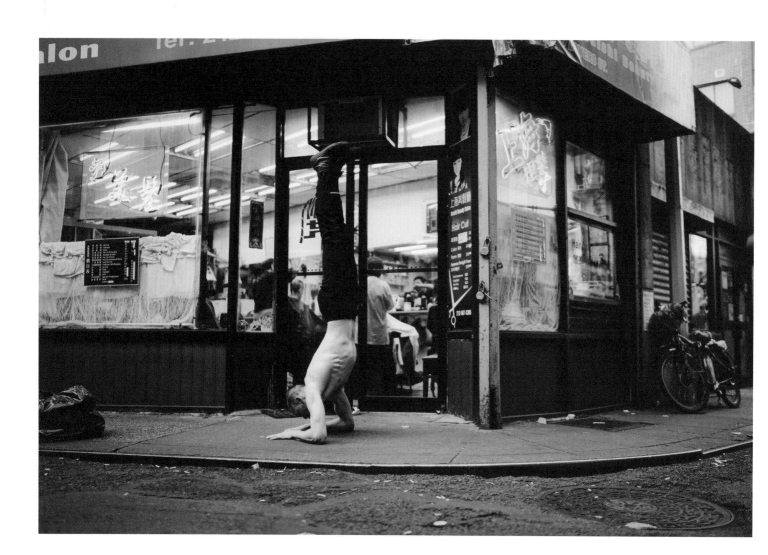

grains (quinoa, wild rice), and on the fifth day I added back dairy. At this point I was still all good—I had a ton of energy, felt full after meals, and was superproud of myself for not having a doughnut. On my eighth day I added sugar back into the mix. That's when things got weird for me. I had a tiny cupcake after dinner (because look at me, I am healthy AF and I deserve this), and I woke up the next morning with a hangover. I am talking a *massive* headache.

The cupcake was the low point in my personal nutrition journey. I had a mild meltdown . . . Did this mean I could never have a cupcake again? Or worse, did it mean I could never have sugar again? *Why me?* I thought about giving up, but balanced nutrition is a lot like yoga—it takes practice and perseverance to find what really works for you. For me, it's like this: sugar is my bad food. Through more trial and error, I found that I had no problem tolerating fruit, honey, or any other naturally occurring sugar, but I do have issues with refined sugar. I'm not here to bore you with a list of things I can and cannot eat, but the story of my nutrition journey contains a lesson that applies to everyone: *You need to figure out what works for your body.* No one else can tell you what you can or cannot eat. Listen to your body and see what it needs from you. If you're unsure or worried, consult a doctor or a professional nutritionist for some guidance. But don't ever stop trusting your understanding of your own body; especially once you begin a yoga practice, you'll be amazed at how well you understand your physical being.

And listen, even after all that exploration and my nutrition studies, I am not "perfect" by any means. I still allow myself to have that cupcake or piece of cake every now and then, because what would life be without some funfetti cake? I used to be really hard on myself if I was not following a diet to the T—but what's the point of being that rigid? Give yourself a break and practice the self-love we talked about earlier (see page 17). As long as you are doing the best you can, and working toward *your* goals and *your* happiness, you are on the right path.

EATING AND DRINKING BEFORE AND AFTER YOGA (...ESPECIALLY HOT YOGA)

Nutrition in general is about maintaining balance and finding what works best for your body. But there are some situations where it's good to be a little more methodical about your approach. It is always a good idea to go into a workout with something in your belly, especially since you will need that extra energy to get through it. But you need to be smart about what you eat—you definitely don't want to be burping up that little snack of guac and chips you decided on. Go with a snack that's filling but light, and always something that you know sits well in your system. It is great to have protein in your body to keep your energy up—anything from nuts to a protein shake would be a great choice.

Keeping hydrated is also an important component of your workout. When it comes to hot yoga in particular (which we practice in the studio at Y7, and which I highly encourage you to try out), there are lots of different schools of thought about how much water to drink and when to drink it. I always tell my clients that it is important to be hydrated, and you should begin drinking a good amount of water an hour before class. As you get closer to class—or any other serious workout—you will want to taper off your water consumption. It is superuncomfortable to go into poses like Forward Fold, or any sort of twist, if your belly is full of liquid. Take tiny sips throughout class as needed, but avoid gulping down an entire bottle—if you take in too much liquid, you will not be happy. After class your motto needs to be: rehydrate, rehydrate, rehydrate. Literally, just go for it. Drink all of the water.

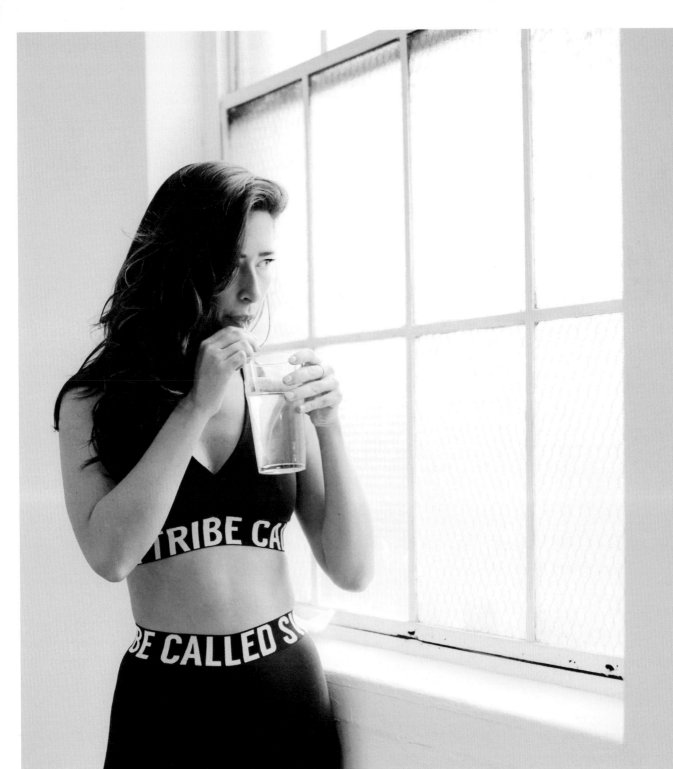

CARING FOR YOUR BODY

Self-care is so important. It's something we often think of as "treating ourselves," but really, those things that seem like indulgences are a key component of cultivating well-being. Maybe you're a little skeptical, but think about it: If you are not at your best, how can you possibly give to anyone else? Caring for your body isn't just one thing; it's a multitude of things. It is physical activity, having a well-rounded diet, and taking time for yourself.

A yoga practice is an amazing way to care for your body. You are engaging in a physical activity, focusing on your body, and working on quieting the mind and blocking out those negative thoughts and judgments. And what is so special about yoga is that it can be practiced often, even every day if you want to. If you do choose to practice every day that is *amazing*, though I would encourage you to ease your way into such a rigorous schedule and mix up your practice with different types of yoga.

As with everything in this chapter, it's all about that balance. I personally always take one day each week completely off from any physical workout. I like to give my body a chance to relax, and it's also important for me to know that can I have a day, or even two, off without losing the momentum I have built (or gaining fifteen pounds). For other people, taking days off can feel like a setback or like they aren't trying hard enough. Those kinds of negative thoughts can be tough to bounce back from, so try a few different options to see what sort of schedule makes sense in your life. And if you do lose momentum, don't lose heart. Get back into the groove with something low-key—you don't have to go in for a two-hour workout the day after your setback, just do *something*. Get on the treadmill for twenty minutes, go for a walk, do a quick ab workout, or find something to motivate you again. When I'm not feeling motivated, I like to book a class with friends so that I will be held accountable if I bail. It's great to have that support system around when you are feeling less than 100 percent, and the sense of camaraderie helps make working out feel less goal-oriented and more fun.

In addition to giving some love to your physical body, it's important to take care of your mental health as well. Make sure that you are doing things for yourself that make you happy. Get that facial, get that weekly mani/pedi—I know it seems like an unnecessary indulgence, but if those things make you happy, then you should do them! That small act of doing something just for yourself can have an amazing mental payoff; it's a little reminder that your well-being is worth tending to. My mani/pedi ritual is

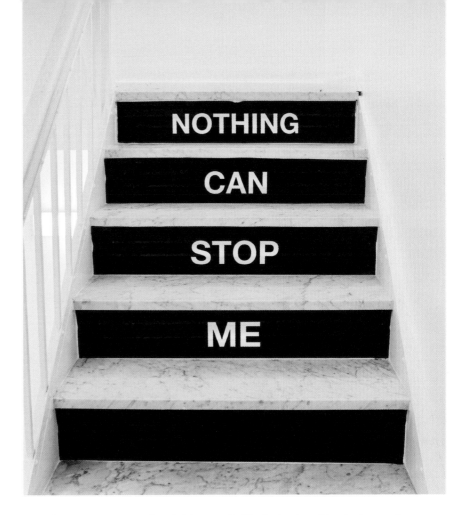

very important to me. It might sound silly, but when I look down at my fingers and see perfectly manicured nails, I know that I look confident and presentable even if I feel less so that day. And that knowledge helps to balance out my negative feelings, giving me the boost I need to regain some of my positivity and confidence. That's just my ritual; for you it may be something else. The point is, honor yourself by carving out the time to do something wholly for you that will enhance your outlook and self-esteem even during the times when you're busy or overwhelmed. Why would you deny yourself something that makes you happy? That's certainly not what we believe at Y7.

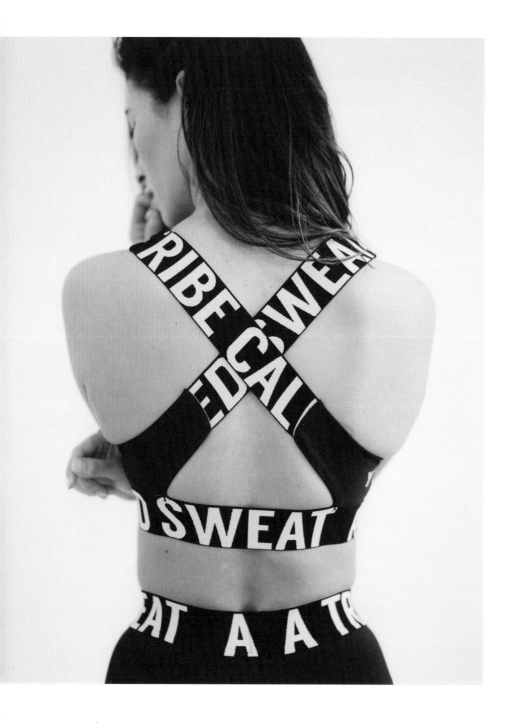

RECIPES

Fueling your body is a key component of performing well and feeling your best. There are so many wonderful cookbooks and blogs out there that provide amazing inspiration for home cooking, which I try to work into my routine on a regular basis. Don't get me wrong, I love the healthy, satisfying options that are out there—especially in my home bases of New York and LA—but making food for yourself is a great habit to get into. Not only are you able to completely control what goes into your food, but you're also finding one more way to set aside time that says "I'm worth that extra effort." Here are some of my favorite recipes for making at home, from breakfast to cocktail time (if that's more your speed, skip ahead to page 165).

Breakfast

Breakfast isn't always the easiest meal of the day to get excited about—who wants to get up extra early just to cook? But putting something into your body early in the day helps to jump-start your metabolism and is the fuel you need to be the badass I know you are. These breakfasts are easy and satisfying to start your day on the right foot.

Overnight Oats with Berries

INGREDIENTS

¼ cup quick oats

½ cup almond milk (or any other milk you desire; I like to use unsweetened almond)

¼ cup blueberries

¼ cup raspberries

1 tbsp chia seeds

½ tsp pure vanilla extract

This is one of my favorite breakfasts, and it's one of the easiest things you can make. This is a no-fuss recipe you can literally grab and go. And best of all, the oats are a great base (and friendly for any of you who are gluten-free). You can change up the recipe depending on your mood—add different toppings or spices based on your own preferences or what's in season. I always favor berries over the cinnamon or honey versions of overnight oats, but when you're making this, you should do you! Here is my go-to version.

METHOD

Mix all the ingredients together in a mason jar or other container, cover, and let everything sit overnight in the fridge. In the morning, open the top of the jar and eat first thing. Just kidding! If early morning eating isn't your style, you can throw the jar in your bag and eat it at the office, on the subway, or anywhere else you might want—it travels well.

Breakfast Bowl (So Hard)

INGREDIENTS

¼ cup cooked quinoa (either make your own by following package directions, or buy precooked quinoa at your local grocery or health foods store)

¼ cup tomato, chopped (approximately one small tomato)

1 scallion, chopped

a few leaves of fresh basil, roughly chopped

½ avocado, diced

1 tbsp olive oil

1 handful of baby spinach

2 eggs (scrambled, fried, or poached—but who has the time or the skill for that—however you like them will work fine here)

Salt and pepper, to taste

Fun fact: I like to have what I call "base foods" on hand in my kitchen at all times. That means cooked quinoa or wild rice, mixed greens, chopped kale, eggs, and broth. I am not a huge meal prepper (I've tried this popular technique, but it really hasn't worked out for me thus far), but I find having a few items at my disposal makes being healthy in the kitchen so much easier. This breakfast bowl takes a base of cooked quinoa and layers on some of my favorite toppings to create a really satisfying meal that sustains me all through the morning.

METHOD

I know that the ingredients list for this recipe makes it seem like there are a lot of things happening—but there really isn't much work involved, and the components blend together super well. (And remember, you already have your quinoa cooked from your meal prep, so look at you go!) In a bowl (whatever size you use for cereal or soup), combine the quinoa, chopped tomato, scallion, basil, and avocado with a tablespoon of olive oil. Set aside. In a small nonstick pan place a large handful of spinach and cook over medium heat, just until the spinach begins to wilt. Once the spinach is done cooking (this process should only take two or three minutes, literally), spoon it over the quinoa mixture. In the same pan you used to sauté your spinach, make your eggs—remember, choose whichever preparation you like best. Once your eggs are cooked to your preferred doneness, place them in the bowl, on top of the spinach. Salt and pepper your final product to taste. Voilá! You are basically a gourmet chef, who has created a well-balanced breakfast full of protein, whole grains, and healthy fats. *Look at you go!*

Lunch

I am pretty much the queen of the desk lunch. I know everyone says you should take a break from your desk and go have lunch, but as the owner of a growing business, I've never really done that. These are lunches that you can make ahead and eat at your desk, without feeling sad.

Tuna Salad Lettuce Wraps

INGREDIENTS

1 tsp yellow mustard

1 tbsp light mayonnaise

¼ chopped white onion

1 tsp fresh parsley, chopped

¼ cup celery chopped

handful of dried cherries

1 can albacore tuna (packed in water), drained

Salt and pepper, to taste

4 leaves of butter lettuce

I like to keep my lunches light, yet satisfying. These lettuce wraps bring in protein, some good veggies, and a little bit of tart sweetness from the dried cherries. And the wraps make it feel special—because who doesn't want to feel a little fancy while they're eating lunch?

METHOD

In the bottom of a bowl, mix the mustard, mayo, onion, parsley, celery, and cherries. You want to get all those flavors melded together before adding in the tuna. Mix in the tuna, stir well to combine, and add salt and pepper to taste.

If you're packing this lunch, put the tuna in a container, and take four leaves of butter lettuce for your wraps. To assemble, place one quarter of the mixture on each leaf of lettuce, tuck the leaves around the tuna, and enjoy!

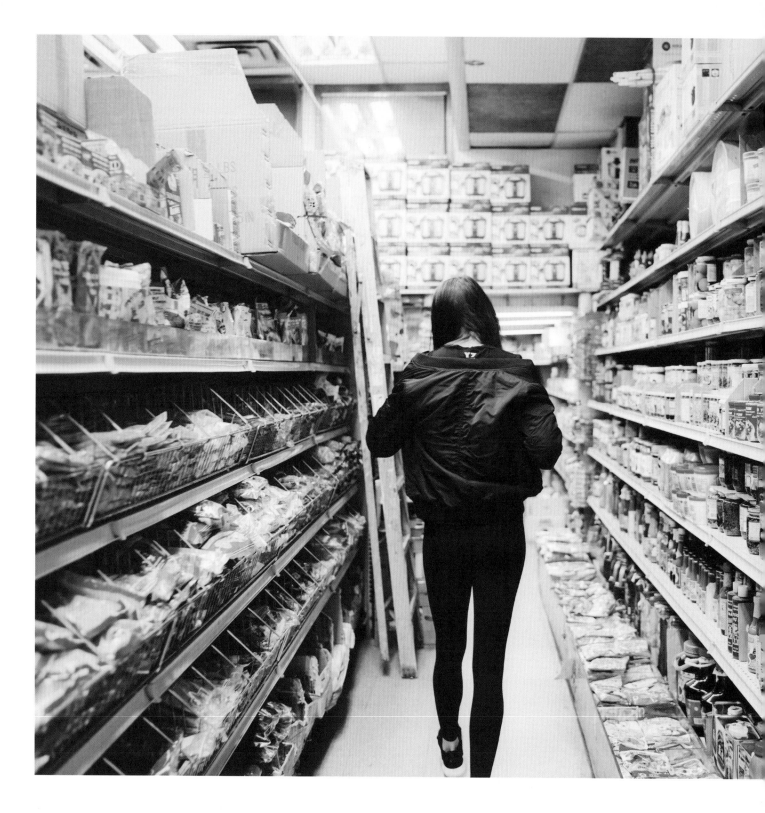

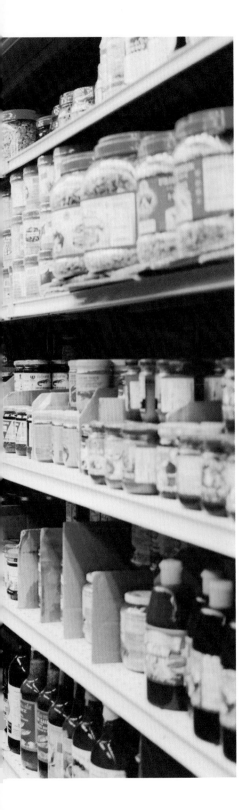

Caprese Salad on Crack

INGREDIENTS

1 cup fresh mozzarella (you can either chop up a larger piece, or buy the small balls of mozzarella that come packed in water)

2 medium tomatoes, chopped

2 tbsp olive oil

1 tbsp balsamic vinegar

2 tbsp chopped basil

¼ lb prosciutto, sliced

½ avocado, sliced

salt and pepper, to taste

I love a classic caprese salad as much as the next girl. But sometimes I feel like the traditional combo needs a little extra oomph to make it a truly satisfying lunch. In this salad I amp up the protein and healthy fats by adding in prosciutto and avocado.

METHOD

Mix all of the ingredients together in a medium-sized bowl, and salt and pepper to taste. Either eat right away, or place in a Tupperware for easy transportation and on-the-go eating.

Dinner

Dinner is the best meal of the day, in my opinion. You can really show off your skills in the kitchen at dinner, and for those of us with busy work schedules, it's usually the only meal of the day when we can really sit down and relax. I like to keep my dinners at home on the healthier side (so I can really enjoy that pizza or pasta when I'm out at a restaurant), but still packed full of flavor.

Garlic Butter Salmon

MAKES 2 SERVINGS

INGREDIENTS

2 tbsp lemon juice

2 cloves garlic, minced

2 tbsp unsalted butter

¼ tsp Italian seasoning blend (you can find this in any major grocery store; in a pinch, substitute ⅛ tsp dried oregano and ⅛ tsp dried basil)

¼ tsp crushed red pepper flakes

¼ tsp black pepper

½ tsp salt

1 lb salmon filet, skin removed

1 tbsp fresh parsley, chopped

This dinner uses one of my favorite techniques for cooking salmon—baking in foil. That's how my dad cooks his salmon, and he's always been my hero (in the kitchen and out!), so obviously I'm not going to question his methods. The foil wraps in all of the delicious juices from the marinade and keeps everything really moist. Salmon is incredibly good for you (packed full of those omega-3 fatty acids), and it's always a crowd-pleaser. Double (or triple!) the recipe if you're having company.

METHOD

Preheat the oven to 375°F. Meanwhile, on the stove, place a sauté pan over medium heat. Add in the lemon juice and garlic and gently sauté for a few minutes—you want to allow the lemon juice to reduce by about half, then add one tablespoon of butter. Remove the pan from the heat and stir so that the butter begins to melt but not burn. Place the pan back on the heat for a few seconds and repeat the same process with the second tablespoon of butter. Once the butter has all melted, add in the spices

(Italian seasoning, red pepper, black pepper, salt). Set this mixture aside for the moment.

Prepare a baking sheet for your salmon; lay out a piece of foil that is larger than your salmon on top of the sheet. Place the salmon in the center of the foil, and fold up the edges to create a little "boat" for your fish. Once your boat is ready, brush the salmon with your reserved butter sauce using a silicon or pastry brush (*yum!*). And don't be shy about it—get all of that sauce on there. If you don't have a brush on hand, just spoon the mixture evenly over the filet. Press the sides of your foil boat together, leaving only a small opening at the top—this will allow your steam to escape, keeping your fish moist but not soggy. Place the salmon in the oven and cook for about 12 to 14 minutes, until the fish is a nice orangey pink and the flesh is beginning to flake. Open the foil packet and sprinkle the fresh parsley on top, then return to the oven and allow the salmon to cook for another minute or two, just to crisp the top (keep a close eye on it). Serve immediately! For side dishes, I recommend roasted asparagus (you can just toss asparagus stalks with a little olive oil, salt, and pepper and roast at the same time as the salmon) and some of the quinoa that you have on hand from your meal prep. (Don't you feel prepared and awesome for having that ready to go?)

Beer, Honey, and Lime Chicken

MAKES 4 SERVINGS

INGREDIENTS

⅓ cup honey (I always try to use local, since not only is it tastier, but local honey helps combat seasonal allergies—bonus!)

1 tsp Dijon mustard

¼ cup low sodium soy sauce (any brand is fine, or substitute liquid aminos if you're avoiding soy)

¾ cup dark beer (I like Negro Modelo)

1 tbsp olive oil

3 cloves of garlic, minced

4 chicken breasts (I usually use boneless, skinless breasts for easy prep and cleanup, but you can use any kind you like—just be sure to adjust your cooking time accordingly)

lime wedges, for serving

handful of cilantro, chopped, for serving

This dinner is just so fun. What's not to love about a marinade that includes beer? I enjoy making this chicken all year round, but it especially helps brighten my mood during drab, gray, winter days. The marinade is incredibly versatile, so feel free to use it on any kind of meat you like or even veggies or firm tofu!

METHOD

In the bottom of a large bowl whisk together the honey, mustard, soy sauce, beer, olive oil, and garlic until the mixture has an even consistency. Place your chicken in the bowl and cover it in this beautiful mixture. Move the bowl to the fridge, and let the chicken marinate for at least two hours and up to overnight.

When you're ready to eat, cook the chicken however you like it best. This marinade is so versatile, it works with any cooking method—you can grill it (on medium-high heat for about 5 to 6 minutes per side), you can bake it (at 350°F for about 30 minutes), you can make it in a pan (in a nonstick skillet, preheated to medium high, and then cooked over medium heat for 8 to 12 minutes, turning occasionally). The world is your oyster in terms of cooking method!

Once the chicken is cooked, squeeze a wedge of lime over the top of each breast and sprinkle with chopped cilantro. Since this chicken dish is packed with so much flavor, I like to serve it with just a simple mixed green and kale salad, dressed in olive oil and balsamic vinegar.

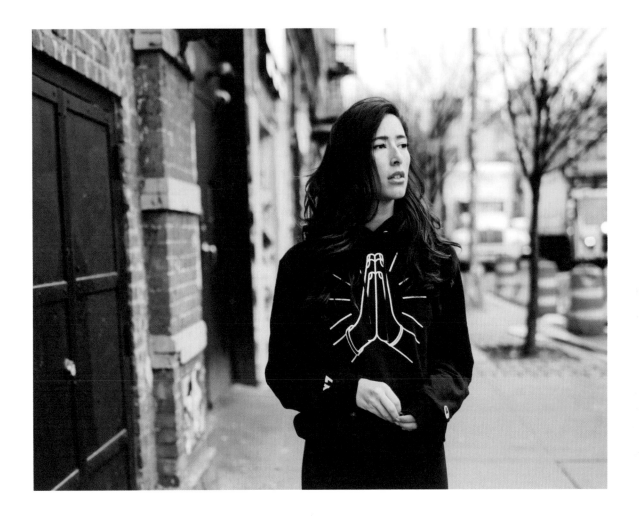

Snack

Whether it's before your workout or in the middle of a long afternoon, I'm all about a healthy snack. There are a lot of great snacks out there that don't require any work at all—raw nuts, cut-up fruit, and veggies with hummus are all excellent options. But sometimes you want a snack that's a little more exciting, but still leaves you feeling light, healthy, and energized. Don't worry—I've got you covered.

Cauliflower Breadsticks

INGREDIENTS

2 cups riced cauliflower (you can create your own riced cauliflower by using a handheld cheese grater or food processor; you can also buy pre-riced cauliflower (fresh or frozen) from grocery stores like Trader Joe's or Whole Foods)

¼ cup shredded Parmesan cheese

1 egg

1 tbsp dried oregano

1 tbsp dried basil

salt and black pepper to taste

This recipe makes the most delicious, addictive cauliflower "breadsticks." They deliver all the taste without feeling like too much of an indulgence. And they're a big hit when you're entertaining! Bonus: this recipe can also be used to make a crust for a gluten-free pizza!

METHOD

Preheat your oven to 425°F. Microwave your riced cauliflower for 4 minutes with a steam cover; if you don't have a steam cover, place your riced cauli-flower in a shallow bowl, add a tablespoon or two of water, and cover with plastic wrap. Drain the cooked cauliflower in a strainer—you want to make sure that you remove as much of the moisture as possible (feel free to place the cauliflower in a tea towel and squeeze out the water over the sink if your batch seems a little waterlogged). Transfer the drained cauliflower to a bowl and add the rest of the ingredients, stirring well. Spread this mixture out on a parchment paper–lined baking pan in whatever shape you want—a rectangle, circle, heart, you name it. Have some fun with your food! Bake for at least 20 minutes, or until the cauliflower mixture reaches your desired level of crispness. Allow to rest for a few minutes, until the cauliflower is cool enough to touch. Cut the mixture into strips and serve immediately with your favorite condiments—I prefer ranch dressing for these (because I am from Michigan, and that is what we do), but they're just as delicious with ketchup, aioli, or tomato sauce.

Cocktails

If you haven't caught on by now, the Y7 approach to health and wellness isn't about deprivation—it's about balance. And for me that means enjoying some cocktails now and then! My favorite spirit is tequila, partly because I love the flavor, and partly because relative to other spirits it's actually pretty good for you. Not only is tequila a gluten-free spirit (for those of you with celiac or a gluten intolerance), it also contains fewer congeners than dark spirits or red wine (congeners are the nasty particles that contribute to your hangovers). Just remember one thing: avoid tequilas labeled "reposado" or "mixto," as these will often contain corn syrup or residues that can undercut the benefits of the agave.

Mescal Chill

INGREDIENTS

¼ cup diced cucumber, muddled

4–6 mint leaves

½ oz freshly squeezed lime juice (from about ½ a lime)

1 tsp agave nectar

2 oz mescal

Think of mescal as tequila's smokier, more mysterious cousin. It's still made from agave, but the rules governing what mescal can be distilled from are a little less strict than those for tequila. If you're a fan of whiskey, it's definitely worth giving mescal a try!

METHOD

Fill a tall cocktail glass with ice and set it aside. Muddle the cucumber and mint together at the bottom of a cocktail shaker, using a pestle or the back of a spoon. Once combined, pour in the remaining ingredients and shake vigorously for 15 seconds. Strain the mixture into the ice-filled glass, and stir well. Garnish with a lime wedge and enjoy!

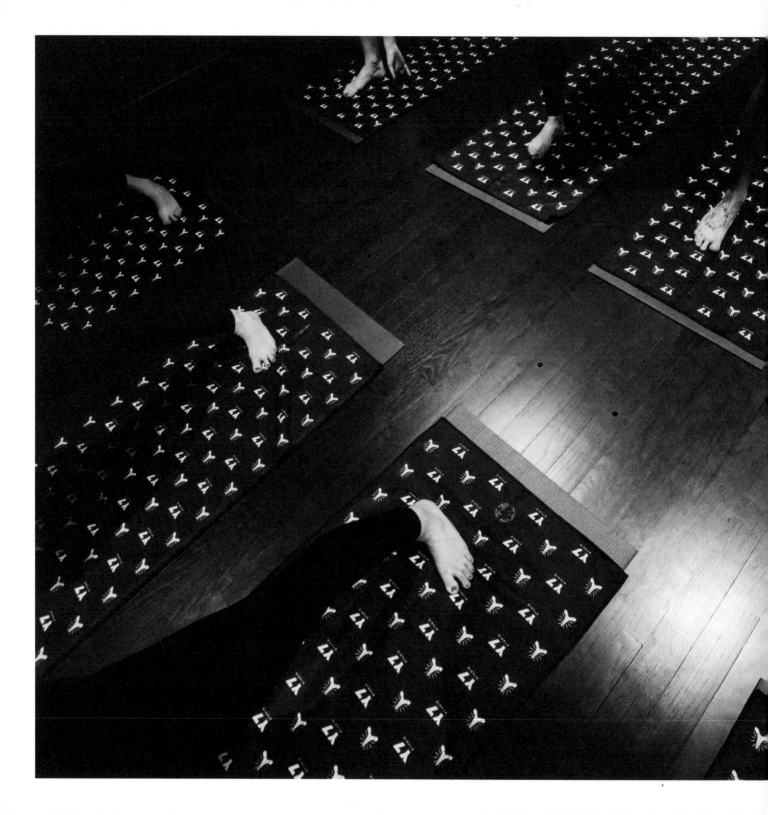

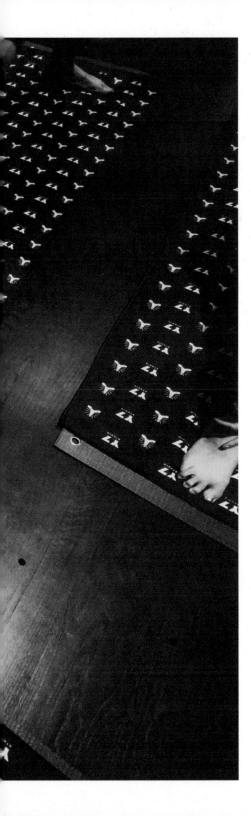

Sarah's Go-To

This is my favorite drink—it is easy, delicious, and exactly what I'm looking for after a long day on the mat. It doesn't have an official name because I made it up on the fly one day; it's more about a method than strict measurements. Customize it with your favorite additions to turn it into your own go-to drink.

INGREDIENTS

Ice

Blanco tequila

Grapefruit sparkling water (La Croix is my favorite brand)

Freshly squeezed lime juice

METHOD

This drink doesn't require specific measurements—it can adapt to the vessel you're using. Fill a glass (like a highball or a mason jar) with ice, then pour in blanco tequila until it reaches the halfway point. Pour in your sparkling grapefruit water until it reaches just below the top of the glass. Add a squeeze of fresh lime juice, stir, and *enjoy.*

NOURISHING YOUR MIND

There is nothing simpler than meditation. As Sri Sri Ravi Shankar, one of our time's most prominent meditation teachers, shares, meditation is the art of doing nothing. At the same time, there are few things more misunderstood. At Y7, we believe that meditation doesn't have to be a massive commitment, and it doesn't have to be done in a particular way. Just like with your yoga practice and your lifestyle, the important thing with meditation is finding what works best for you.

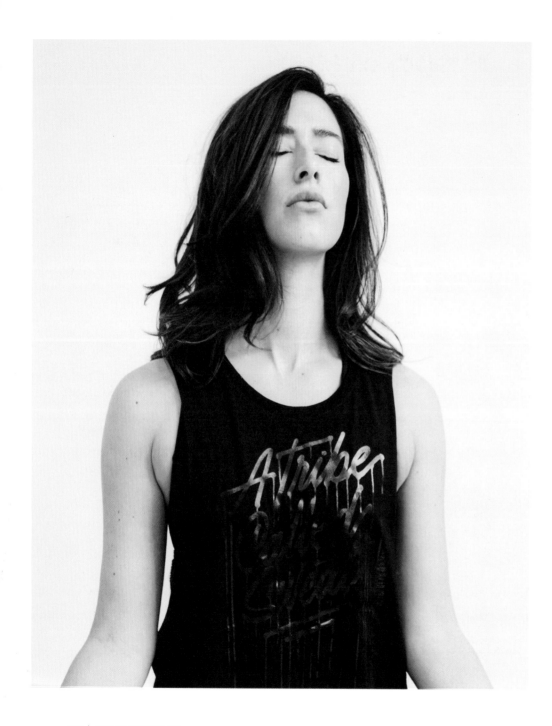

Meditation is simply being with yourself and resting deeply and consciously. It is a small act, but something that can take as few as fifteen minutes of your time delivers big results. When the mind is clear, there is a great difference in our perception, in our happiness, and in our quality of life. Meditation is also about carving out time for yourself—time to connect your body and mind and to refocus your energies. When I started meditating, it didn't take long to notice that I was calmer and more at ease, even with what would otherwise be nerve-racking situations. And I've seen the same benefits for so many of our students at Y7—people who are working hard to balance jobs, social lives, and side hustles, without losing a sense of calm in their lives.

MEDITATION

By Mahadevi Michelle Martini,
creator of the HeavilyMeditated Workshop at Y7 Studio.

We've worked with Mahadevi Michelle Martini—one of our Y7 Artists and a badass meditation teacher—to offer our signature HeavilyMeditated Workshops at Y7 Studios. As you'll read in this chapter, she's the real deal, bringing a holistic understanding of wellness to a modern lifestyle. We're honored to share her techniques in our studios and our book. —Sarah

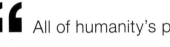

All of humanity's problems stem from man's inability to sit quietly in a room alone."

—*Blaise Pascal*

When we think of meditation, the first things that probably come to mind are its multitude of mental and physical benefits. We might imagine the zen vibes radiating from our pores, as we sit with a gentle smile in perfect posture on a meditation cushion. *Mmmm, bliss!* Right, let's be real. Most of our stabs at meditating probably look a little messier than that idealized image.

Imagine: You have squeezed time in your already packed schedule to sit for meditation. As soon as you close your eyes that never-ending mental check-list starts cycling through your brain. "I have to do *x, y, z*. I don't have time to just sit here. I thought this was supposed to help me relax, and now I feel more anxious than ever! Am I sitting correctly? My back hurts. What's the point?" If this story sounds familiar, you're not alone! Tension, hypertension, stress, and anxiety are some of the most common problems faced in our society today. Stress has become the undercurrent of most of our mental states, and it affects everything we do. Many of us who attempt to meditate start out with these issues. We put forth so much effort in our daily lives just trying to keep our sh*t together, that our minds are trained to be superactive. Tuning inside can be a daunting endeavor to say the least! Consider that when we find stillness in the body, our minds tend to speed up.

How can we stop ourselves from turning the wheels of anxiety that fixate on the things that we *should* be doing while we sit to meditate, essentially doing nothing? It isn't always easy, but it's so important. When we are able to ease the tensions in life, finding emotional balance, we gain a much greater freedom. We are able to do less, because the decisions we make have much more impact. We work "smart" instead of "hard" because we are tapping into our greatest potential. Our nervous systems are balanced, and we have a greater opportunity for healing and overall success.

Our tendency toward anxiety is a natural thing. When our mammalian brains were developing, the sympathetic nervous system was an integral tool in keeping us safe. The fight or flight response is a classic for a reason. When a predator or other danger approached our ancestors, their brains flooded with cortisol to meet the challenge at hand. Our conundrum now is that the evolution of our brains hasn't exactly kept speed with the evolution of modern culture. With the addition of *perceived* stress into our lives—like career pressure, personal relationships, technology, and traffic—the brain finds it more efficient to stay in the sympathetic system, cranking out those fight or flight hormones. This means our stress and cortisol levels are higher than ever. We are missing out on the gems of the parasympathetic system, which facilitates the processes of rest and reflection.

Stemming back over 3,500 years, the ancient Indian roots of meditation have evolved into a staple of the majority of today's religions around the

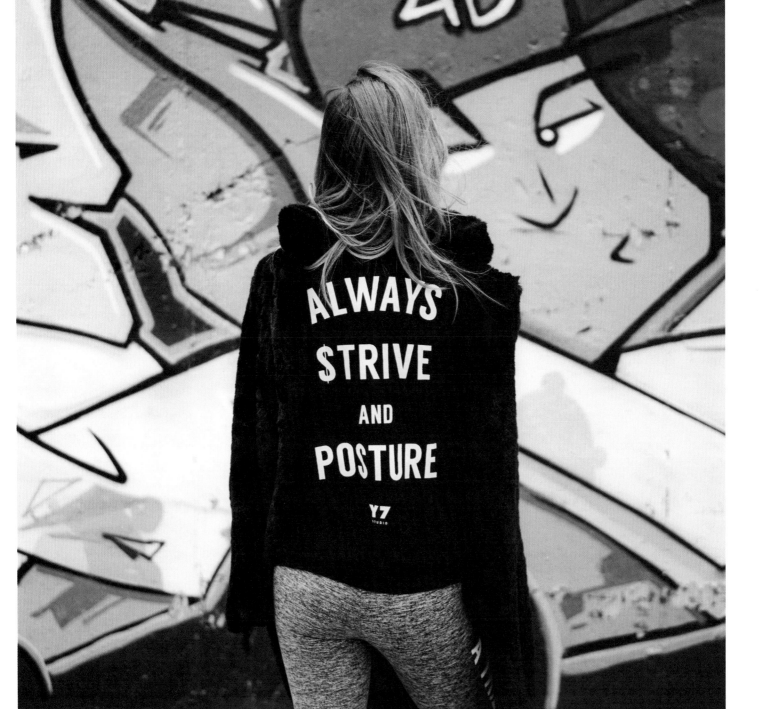

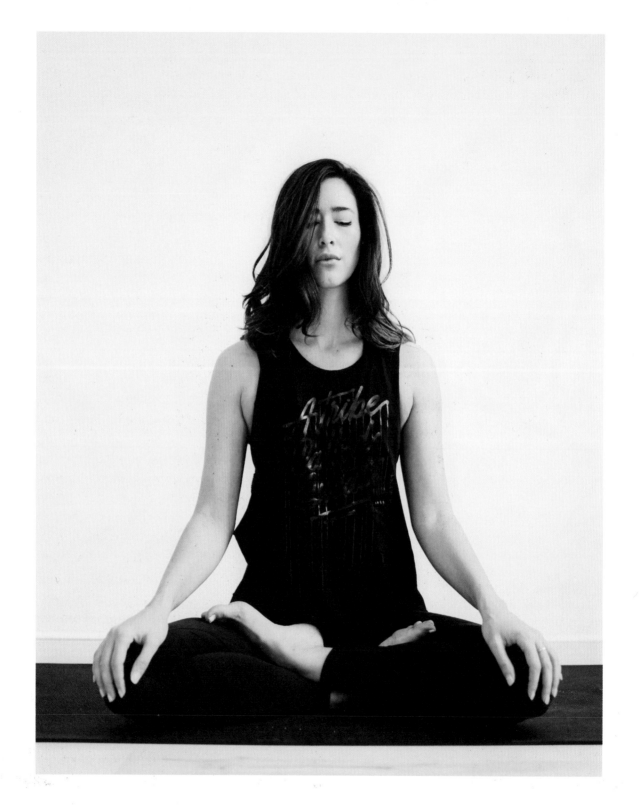

globe. Although it has traditionally been used as a spiritual practice, meditation by no means has to be. Meditation isn't about praying to some foreign or familiar god. The primary premise of meditation is to relax. Our aim is not so much forcing the mind to be still, but rather dissolving resistance to whatever comes up. We learn to allow the body to breathe into whatever shows up—first in our meditative seat, and then into every situation in our lives. Instead of running or reacting when something unpleasant comes up, can we breathe into the moment and show up on a deeper level? This relaxation response, activated by meditation, allows us to tap into deep healing on a mental level, decreasing activity in the sympathetic nervous system and allowing the healing of the parasympathetic system to kick in. Meditation boasts benefits such as significant improvement in mental focus, vitality, peace of mind, and elevated perspective, just to name a few of the hundreds. So, how do we get started?

To begin a regular meditation practice it is important to create a sacred space. It doesn't need to be a fancy altar or adorned with anything in particular, though if doing those things will get you in the best head space, go right ahead. The important thing is to find somewhere quiet and comfortable where you can sit undisturbed for the length of your meditation. Your special space should include a place for you to sit that supports proper posture. Remember that your spine should act like an antenna— straight and tall, but not too rigid, allowing the energy to flow. Whichever seat you choose should be comfortable and supportive. You may sit in a flat-backed chair with your feet on the floor and a cushion bracing the lower back to keep you comfortably erect. A more traditional option is to sit in **Easy Pose**—a cross-legged position, propped up on a pillow, blanket, or cushion. Place your prop under your hips so that they are elevated a few inches above the knees. Also take care to support under the knees, so every part of your base feels at ease and grounded. The aim here is to initiate the relaxation response. Set a timer for your desired length of meditation. There are also some really great apps that track your meditation and mentally bring you back to the room with chimes or bells when your time is complete. You might start with five minutes and gradually add a minute a day until you get up to around thirty.

Be honest and compassionate with yourself about where you are in your practice. Five minutes daily is absolutely better than none at all. Once you have set yourself up for success in the external space, it is time to tune in. Be completely open with yourself and have realistic expectations. Be accepting of whatever arises within your meditation. The mind's nature is to fluctuate, and its state changes every day, throughout the day. Love yourself enough to be gentle with your mind and the experience your meditation brings about. No expectations—this is a judgment-free space where you are facilitating healing and getting to know yourself on a deeper level.

Enjoy your time and have an observational approach, but try not to take the whole thing too seriously. Allow whatever happens to be just that—an experience. Consider this your mental fitness routine. And just like with your workout, consistency is key, so make a commitment to sit down for at least five minutes a day. Find a time that regularly works best for your schedule so that meditation becomes a routine. The morning is generally the best time, but you may prefer to do it before bed as well. Even better yet, do it both morning and night as your "meditation sandwich."

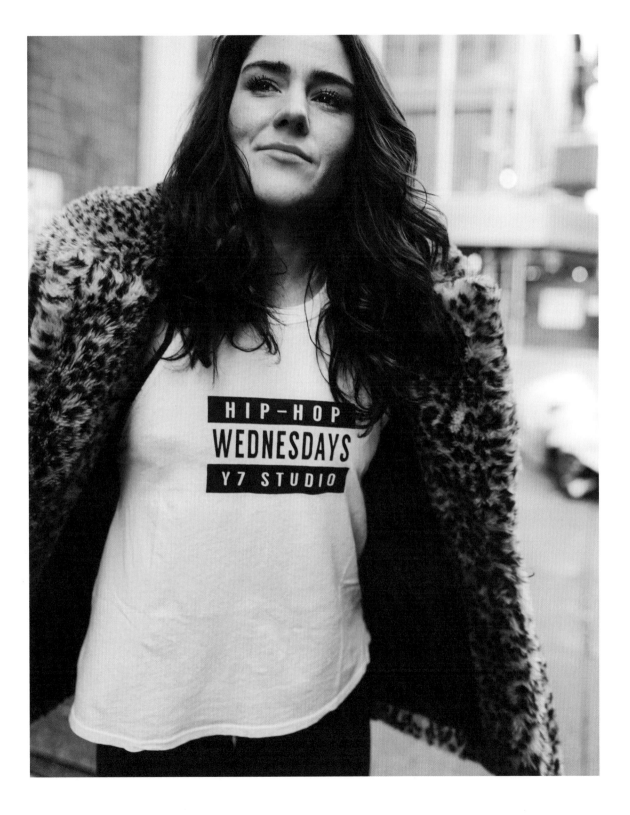

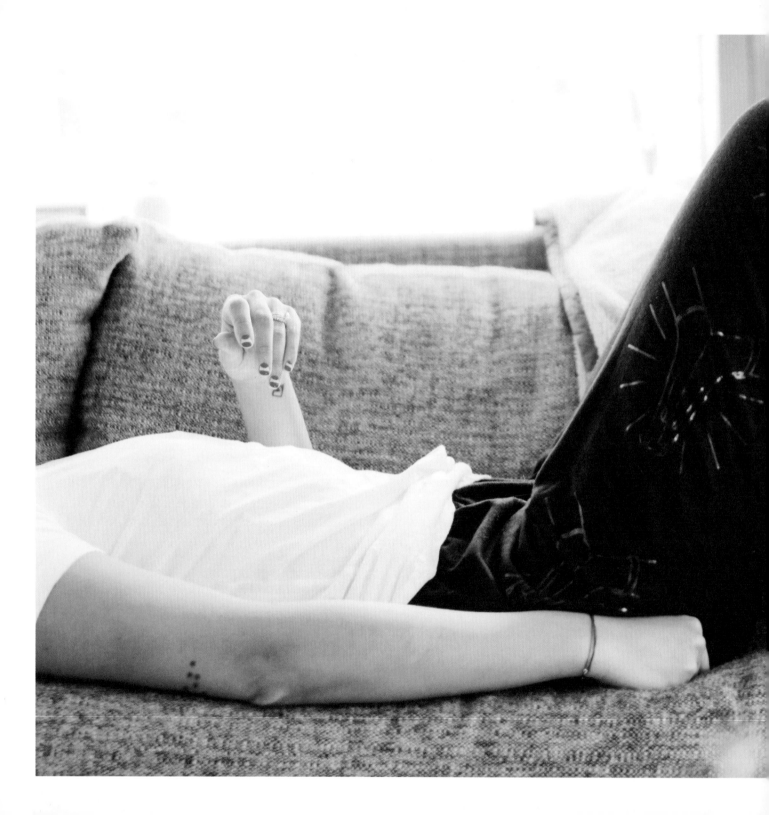

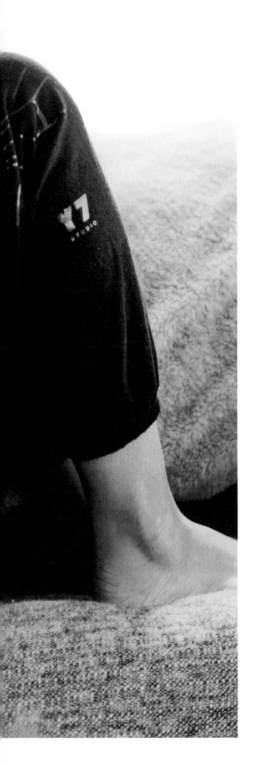

Your Daily Meditation

Close your eyes and start to tune in to your breath. Without judgment, notice the depth of your breath. Notice its pace. Tune in to the temperature of the breath. Maybe you notice the inhale is slightly cooler than the exhale. Try to make each breath a little slower and a little deeper than the one before, without straining the lungs. Starting the Dirgha breath, breathe slowly into the three chambers of the lungs: belly, ribs, and chest. Exhale like a gentle crashing wave from the chest, ribs, and belly. Feel the breath rise thorough the belly, ribs, and chest, and then gently fall through the chest, ribs, and belly. Take about ten rounds of this breath, allowing the mind and heart rate to slow.

Tune in to the sensations of the breath, the feeling of the rib cage widening, the awareness of the lungs expanding from inside the body. Feel gratitude for this precious breath, this nourishing force that is the wind of change in your life. Each inhale fills you up, and each exhale allows you to let go of whatever needs to flow. Employing your mental powers of concentration, use a mantra to focus with the breath. With each inhale silently repeat "let" and with every exhale repeat "go." If any thoughts start to arise, acknowledge them and let them go without dwelling on their contents. Imagine yourself as the infinite and ever-expanding universe. Your thoughts are just shooting stars, energy moving through space. Whenever the mind starts to wander, come back to the breath and back to your mantra.

Meditation in Moments

Meditation doesn't just have to be a seated practice. You can take it with you wherever you go. Ideally, after having a long-standing meditation practice, you will be able to harness its powers through your walking and waking life. Meditation will enable you to use the gifts of serenity and non-attachment to have greater perspective in all that you do.

When you're feeling tense: The next time you feel rushed or stressed, when you are riding the subway or stuck in traffic, take that as an opportunity to come back to the breath. You can do this mini-meditation with your eyes open or closed, alone or surrounded by people. Start with the Dirgha breath and tune in to the sensations of the breath in the body. This breath creates space inside of you and distances you from the perceived stressor in your mind.

Throughout the day: Set an alarm on your phone to go off once or twice a day. Whenever the alarm goes off, use it as a reminder to practice deepening your breath, coming back to your mantra, or finding reasons to be grateful. Gratitude is the best practice to immediately shift yourself into a higher vibration.

Before you eat: Take a couple of deep breaths to allow the breath to feed you. Be grateful for the food and its ability to nourish your body before you eat.

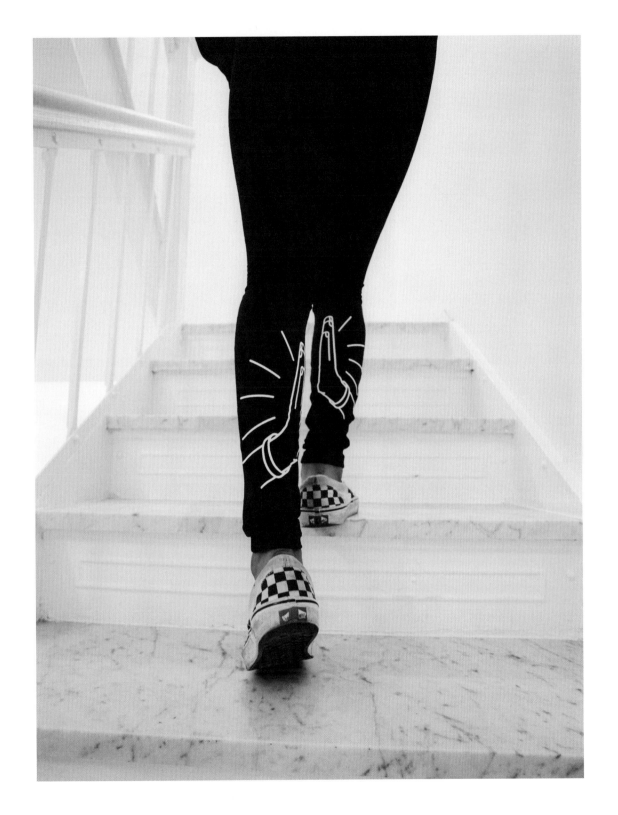

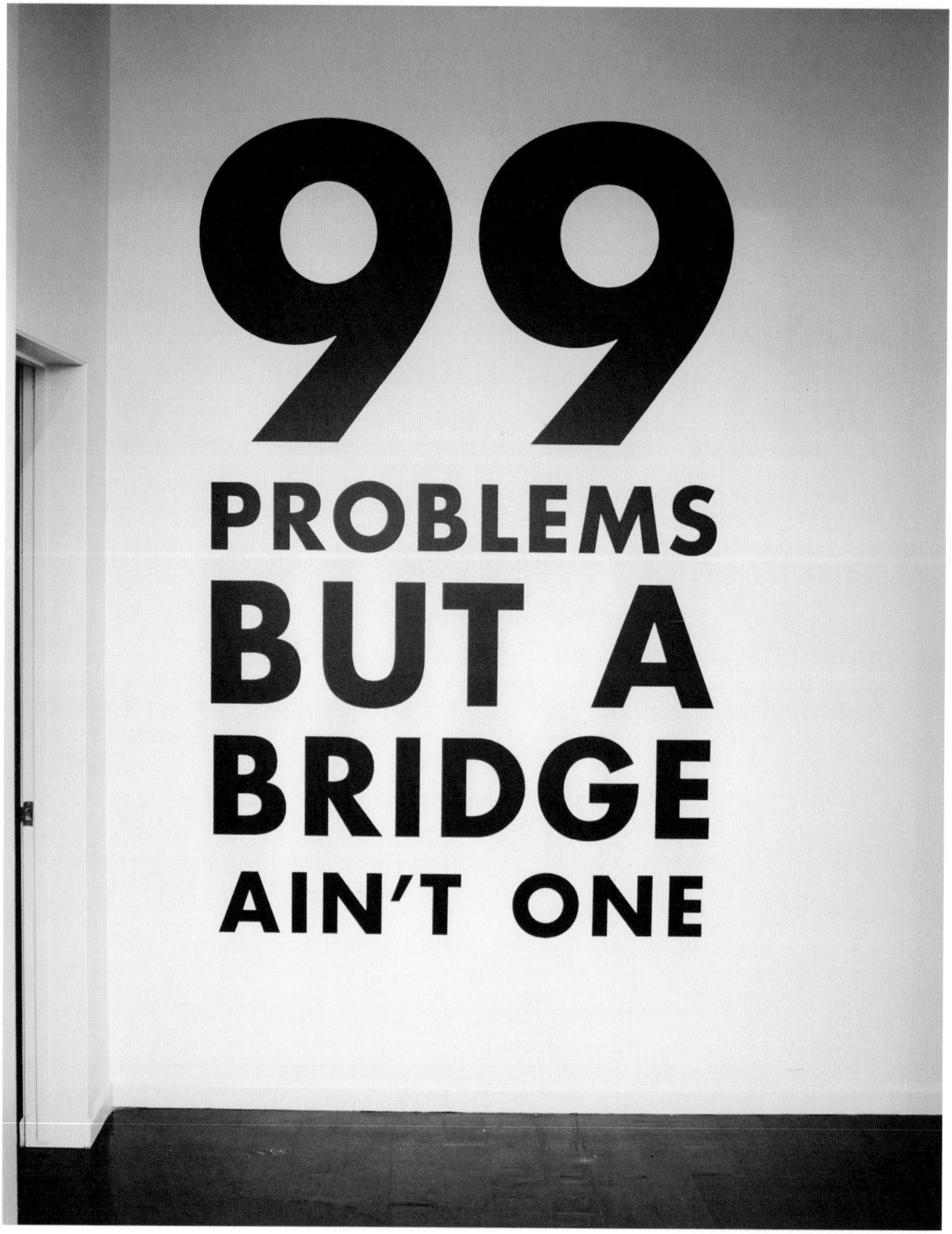
99
PROBLEMS
BUT A
BRIDGE
AIN'T ONE

Yoga Nidra

Sometimes all you need is a quick meditation to ground your mind. But other times, what you want is a deeper, longer practice to recharge you. Yoga Nidra is a form of meditation that works with the powers of the subconscious mind to drop our brain waves into a hypnogogic state . . . or as we like to say, a hypno*yogic* state. This is the state between waking and dreaming, and its applications are more scientific than spiritual. When we look at the brain, we find that the intellectual waking mind is critical and discriminating. Think of it as hard soil. But when we drop into the waves of the subconscious mind, we find that it is extremely receptive and easily impressed with whatever is planted—our soft soil. The suggestions we plant in the subconscious mind can help us remove unwanted tendencies or habits while directing the mind to learn or accomplish anything you can dream of.

In Yoga Nidra, our intention (sankalpa) is the first, last, and most important step. To begin your Yoga Nidra practice, find a comfortable place to lie down. Support beneath the knees and under the head and neck for optimal comfort. We are seeking that hypnoyogic state, so the goal is to fully relax but not fall asleep. Try to remain as conscious as possible as you traverse the bridge from fully awake to the relaxed subconscious mind. This practice is best done guided, so you may want to record yourself with the script I've included below and then play it back to yourself. Allow time for silence in between each of the guided steps.

Guided Yoga Nidra

Close your eyes and feel your body on the floor. Feel your bones melting into the earth, supported by the ground beneath you. Make a commitment not to move for the next half hour.

Sankalpa. Bring your awareness to your intention. Silently repeat it to yourself three times. Envision it in your mind's eye. What does it look like? Who is around? How does it feel?

[PAUSE]

Conscious rotation of the body. Bring your awareness to your: right thumb, right index finger, right middle finger, right ring finger, right pinkie finger. Back of the right hand, center of the right palm. Right wrist, right forearm, right elbow, right upper arm, right armpit, right shoulder, right waist, right hip. Top of the right thigh, right knee, right shin, right ankle, top of the right foot. Right big toe, second toe, third toe, fourth toe, and pinkie toe. Ball of the right foot. Sole of the right foot. Right heel, right calf, right hamstring, right glutes, right back muscles.

Bring your awareness to your: left thumb, left index finger, left middle finger, left ring finger, left pinkie finger. Back of the left hand, center of the left palm. left wrist, left forearm, left elbow, left upper arm, left armpit, left shoulder, left waist, left hip. Top of the left thigh, left knee, left shin, left ankle, top of the left foot. Left big toe, second toe, third toe, fourth toe, and pinkie toe. Ball of the left foot. Sole of the left foot. Left heel, left calf, left hamstring, left glutes, left back muscles. Bring your awareness to your entire right leg. From the toes to the knee to the hip. The entire right leg. Bring your awareness to your entire left leg. From the toes to the knee to the hip. The entire left leg. Bring your awareness to both legs simultaneously. Bring your awareness to your

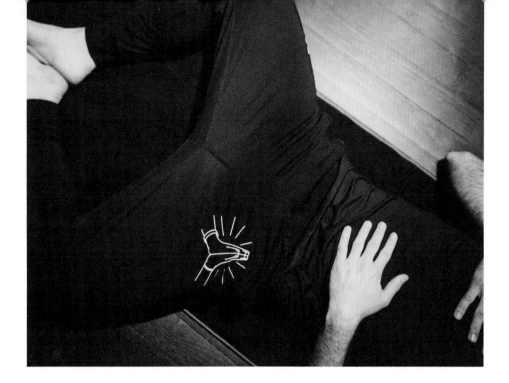

entire right arm. From the fingertips to the elbow to the shoulder. The entire right arm. Bring your awareness to your entire left arm. From the fingertips to the elbow to the shoulder. The entire left arm. Bring your awareness to both arms simultaneously. Bring your awareness to your entire spine, to your entire spine, to your entire spine.

[PAUSE]

Back of the neck, back of the head, crown of the head, forehead, right eyebrow, left eyebrow, third eye center between the eyebrows. Right eyelid, left eyelid, right cheek, left cheek, right nostril, left nostril, tip of the nose. top lip, bottom lip, space where the lips meet. Bring your awareness to your jaw, your tongue, your teeth. Bring your awareness to your entire body, to your entire body, to your entire body. Very good. No sleeping, no sleeping, no sleeping.

[PAUSE]

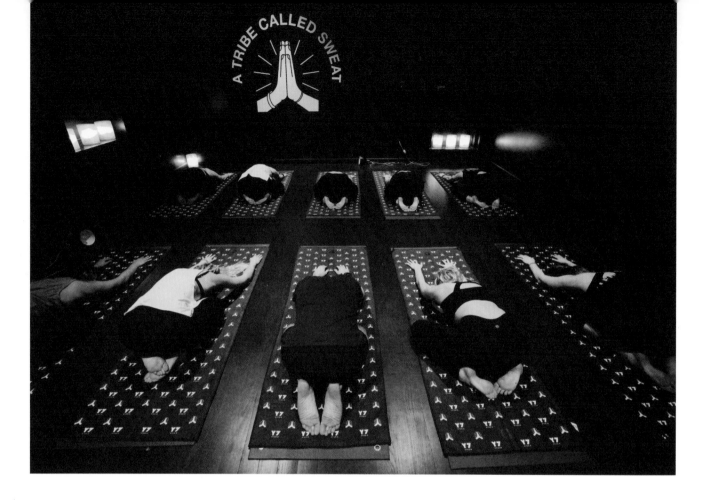

BREATH COUNTDOWN

Bring your awareness to your belly. Notice the rise and fall with every inhale and exhale. Every inhale belly lifts, every exhale belly falls. Counting the breath back from 27, 27 belly lifts (inhale), 27 belly falls (exhale), 26 belly lifts, 26 belly falls. Continue counting back at your own pace. If you get lost, begin again at 27. If you get to 0, begin again at 27.

[LONG PAUSE]

Very good. No sleeping, no sleeping.

OPPOSITES

Feel your body on the floor. Imagine yourself as heavy. So heavy you are immobile. Feel that imminent stillness of the force of gravity. You are heavy, very heavy.

[PAUSE]

Now imagine yourself as light as a feather. You dance like a leaf in the wind. Floating, careless, free.

[PAUSE]

Imagine yourself as hot. You are so hot you are sweating, growing warmer and warmer, feeling the rays of the sun penetrating your skin. You are hot.

[PAUSE]

Now imagine yourself as cold. You are so cold you are shivering. You have goose bumps. You are shivering. You are cold.

[PAUSE]

Bring yourself back to a happy memory.

[PAUSE]

Memory fades, joy remains.

[PAUSE]

JOURNEY

Imagine yourself floating on a cloud. You are suspended in air by this cushiony cloud, slowly floating weightlessly through the sky. You see birds flying in the atmosphere around you. It is around sunset, and the luminous sky is painted with the most magnificent colors. You see other clouds passing by, and you notice certain shapes that they form. These shapes tell a story to your subconscious mind. What is your message?

[LONG PAUSE]

RANDOM IMAGES

Now envision a bird, a waterfall, a tree, a mountain, a lake, a volcano, a deer, a field, a pencil, a dragon, a mirror. See yourself in the mirror. See yourself in the mirror. See yourself in the mirror.

[PAUSE]

THIRD EYE GAZE

Very good. Gaze into your third eye, at the space between your eyebrows. Your center of consciousness. What do you see?

[PAUSE]

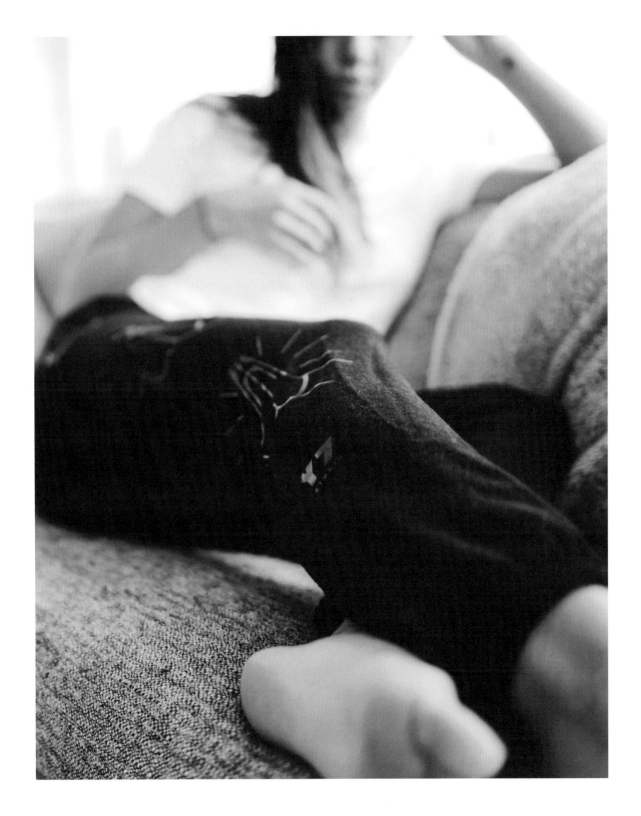

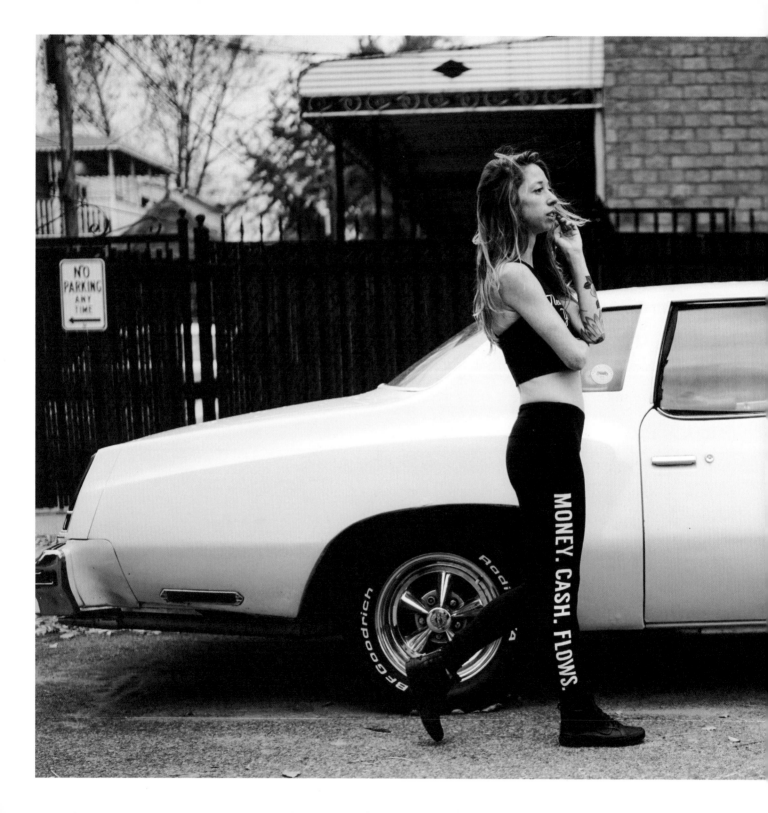

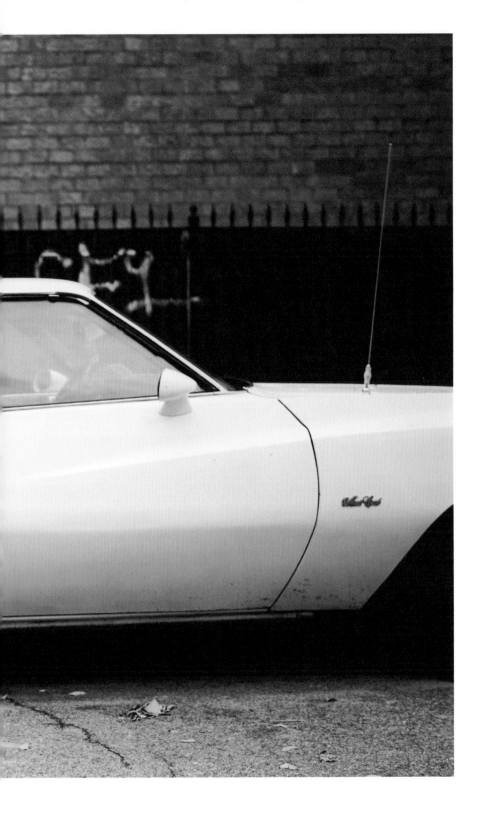

SANKALPA

One last time, bring your awareness to your intention. Silently repeat it to yourself three times. Envision it in your mind's eye. Plant it in the fertile soft soil.

[PAUSE]

Yoga Nidra is now complete. Gently start to deepen the breath in your body. Start to wiggle your fingers and toes. In your own time, gently turn over onto one side, and when you are ready, gently press yourself up to a seat.

AFTERWORD

There are so many things you can take away from this book.

We've discussed our philosophy as Y7, yoga poses that you can incorporate into your workout, building playlists, finding *your* practice, and nourishing your body and spirit. We have touched on different parts of life and how yoga has the ability to not only enhance your physical body, but to bring mental clarity as well. I hope what you have read has inspired you to take up your own practice and make it a part of your everyday life. I hope you start doing Down Dog to Missy Elliott. But above all I hope you've learned how to balance your body and mind while staying honest with yourself and your goals. The Y7 community is not just in the studios. It is everyone who has dared to think differently and push the boundaries of what has been done before.

The light in me sees, honors, and respects the very same light in you. Namaste.

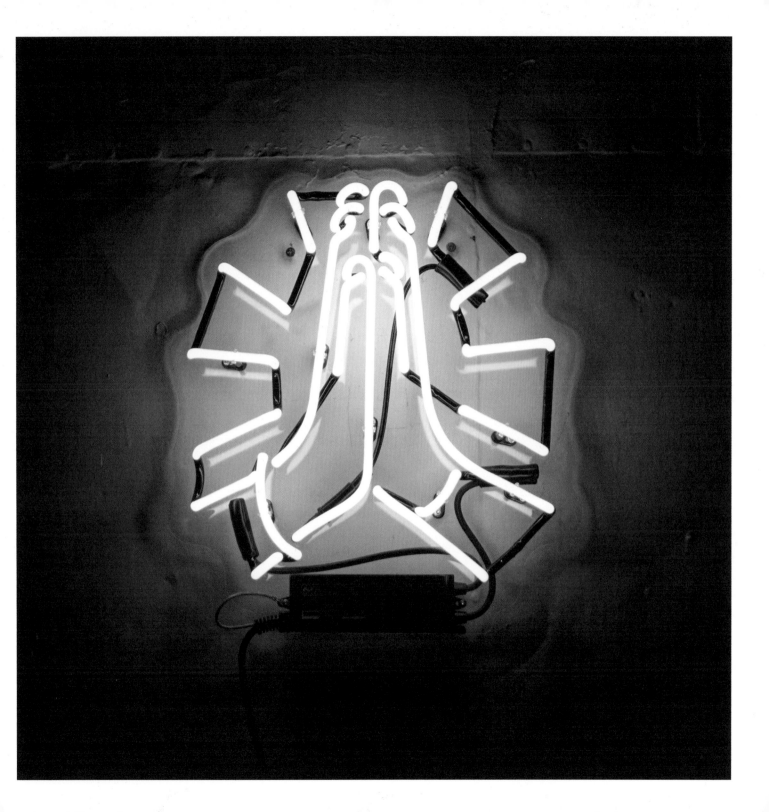

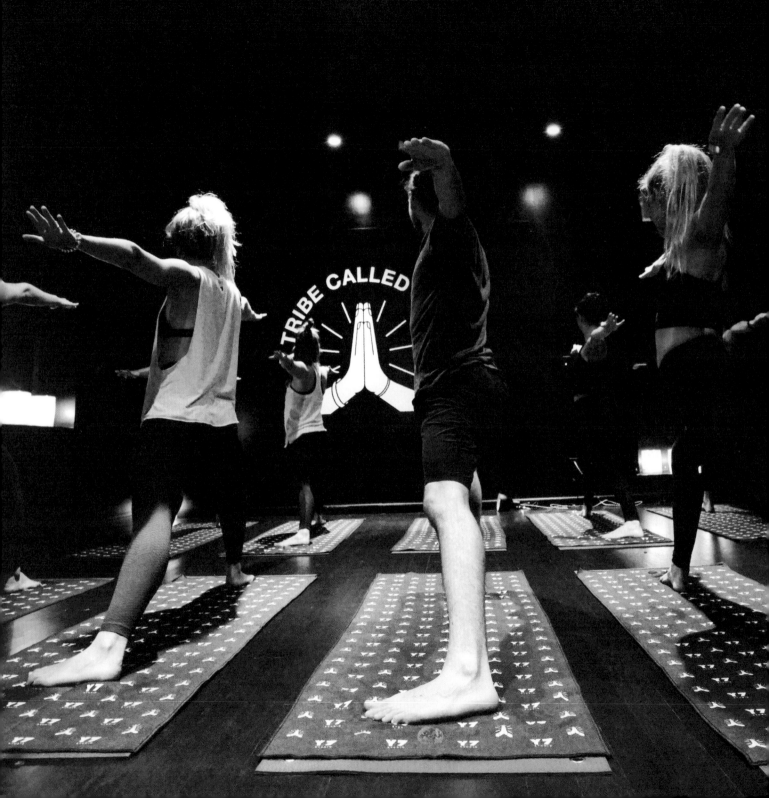

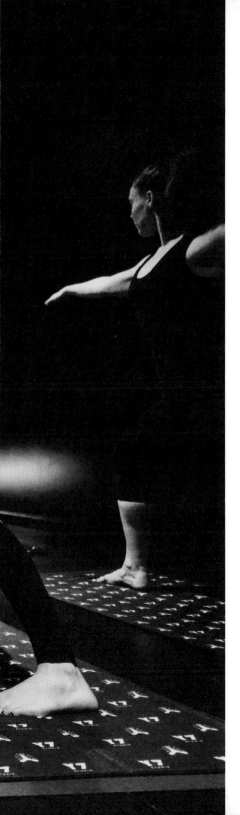

Acknowledgments

Writing this book has been a collective process in every sense. I am so grateful to our tribe—without you this would never have been possible.

Y7's story so far has been unconventional to say the least—and we would not be anything without our clients. Thank you for taking a chance on hip-hop yoga, and for continuing to motivate us to innovate an already inspiring community.

Thank you to our instructors and teaching leadership team, who work endlessly to make the Y7 experience one-of-a-kind. To a particular few of my incredible instructors: Stephanie Laspina, Kristin Lewis, Kristen Nichols, and Michelle Martini, for bringing your voices, perspectives, and passions to the yoga community and beyond.

Thank you to Emily DiDonato for your beautiful spirit, kind words, and for taking the time to share your Y7 experience.

A special thank you to Brad Warsh for the incredible photography, inspiration, and creativity in bringing the Y7 brand alive on these pages. And thank you to designer Ashley Todd for your care in translating our vision into print.

Thank you to my editor Shannon Connors, who helped me every step of the way—your patience and guidance made writing an incredible experience. I could not have done this without your expertise.

Finally, thank you to my husband, cofounder, and partner Mason, for challenging, questioning, and pushing me to be better during the process of it all.

195

Pose Glossary

BALANCING TABLETOP: *Dandayamna Bharmanasana*. Balancing pose that works to build stability within the body. One arm is stretched out long in front of the body and the opposite leg is stretched out long behind.

BOAT POSE: *Navasana*. Core strengthening posture in which the body is in a V shape and you are balancing on your sit bones.

CAT POSE: *Marjaryasana*. Core strengthening pose on hands and knees where the core is pulled in and the spine rounds.

CHAIR POSE: *Utkatasana*. Standing pose that strengthens the core and lower body, the arms extend upward as the knees bend.

CHAIR TWIST: *Parivrtta Utkatasana*. Variation of Chair Pose challenging balance while stretching the spine, shoulders, and chest, with the elbow hooked outside the opposite knee. Also known as Twisted Chair.

CHATURANGA DANDASANA: *Four-Limbed Staff Pose*. Similar to plank pose but with the arms bent to a 90-degree angle, it preps the body for arm balances.

CHILD'S POSE: *Balasana*. Resting pose which stretches the hips, back, and thighs.

CLOSED PRAYER TWIST HIGH LUNGE: *Parivrtta Anjaneyasana*. Standing pose approached from a High Lunge where the elbow is hooked outside the opposite thigh, lengthening the spine and strengthening the legs.

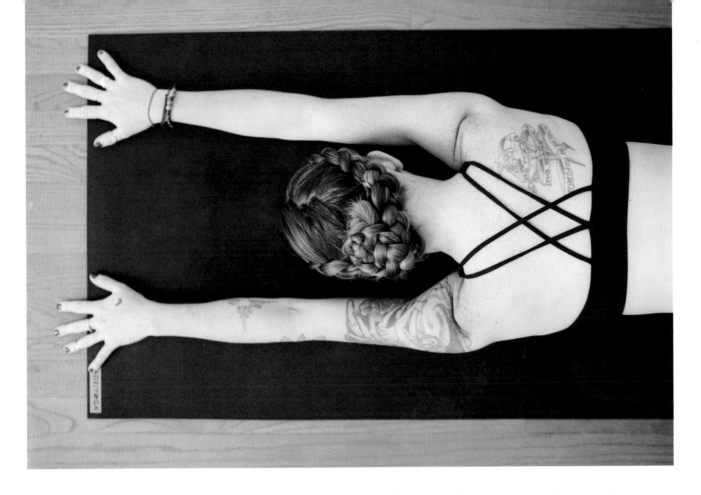

COW POSE: *Bitilasana*. Pose stretching the spine on hands and knees, where the back is arched dropping the stomach toward the ground.

CROW POSE: *Bakasana*. Active balancing pose in which the hands are on the ground, the knees are tucked into the back arms, and the feet are lifted.

DIVERS POSE: *No Sanskrit equivalent*. Standing and balancing pose that works the entire lower body.

DOWNWARD DOG SPLIT: *Eka Pada Adho Mukha Svanasana*. Standing inversion where the leg is raised high above the hip to challenge balance.

DOWNWARD FACING DOG: *Adho Mukha Svanasana*. Pose that builds upper body strength and increases flexibility. Hands and feet are on the ground and the body is in an inverted V shape.

FALLEN TRIANGLE: *No Sanskrit equivalent*. Back-bending and heart opening pose to stretch the front of the body.

FORWARD FOLD: *Uttanasana*. Standing pose that provides a deep stretch for the back of the body.

HALFWAY LIFT: *Ardha Uttanasana*. Standing forward fold variation with the hands on the shins and chest lifted to open the heart.

HALF MOON POSE: *Ardha Chandrasana*. Standing and balancing pose that engages the core and expands the chest.

HIGH LUNGE: *Utthita Ashwa Sanchalanasana*. Standing pose that strengthens the legs and whole lower body.

HIGH LUNGE WITH T-TWIST: *No Sanskrit equivalent*. Standing pose that strengthens the lower body and engages the core with twisting.

LOW BOAT: *Ardha Navasana*. Variation of Boat Pose where the shoulders and legs stay lifted but the lower back is on the ground.

LOW LUNGE: *Anjaneyasana*. Pose that stretches, tones, and lengthens the body.

MOUNTAIN POSE: *Tadasana*. Simple standing pose with the body strong and tall.

PLANK POSE: *Kumbhakasana.* Strengthening and balancing pose that works the arms and core.

PYRAMID POSE: *Parsvottanasana.* Standing side stretch pose that strengthens the legs and stretches the spine, hamstrings, hips, and shoulders.

REVERSE (PEACEFUL) WARRIOR: *Viparita Virabhadrasana.* Standing back-bending pose that provides a deep side stretch.

REVOLVED PEACEFUL WARRIOR: *Parivrtta Viparita Virabhadrasana.* Standing posture that twists the core as it opens the chest.

ROCKSTAR POSE: *Camatkarasana.* Back-bending pose that energizes the whole body and opens the heart.

TABLETOP: *Ardha Purvottanasana.* Beginner's pose in which hands are on the floor under the shoulders and the knees are on the ground under the hips with the body forming the shape of a table.

TRIANGLE POSE: *Trikonasana.* Standing pose that opens the hips and strengthens the ankles, knees, and thighs.

TWISTED CHAIR: *Parivrtta Utkatasana.* Chair pose with a twisted upper body which opens the chest and requires a lot of core strength. Also known as Chair Twist.

UPWARD FACING DOG: *Urdhva Mukha Svanasana.* Back-bending posture that strengthens the arms, shoulders, and wrists.

WARRIOR TWO: *Virabhadrasana B (or II).* Powerful standing posture that opens the hips.

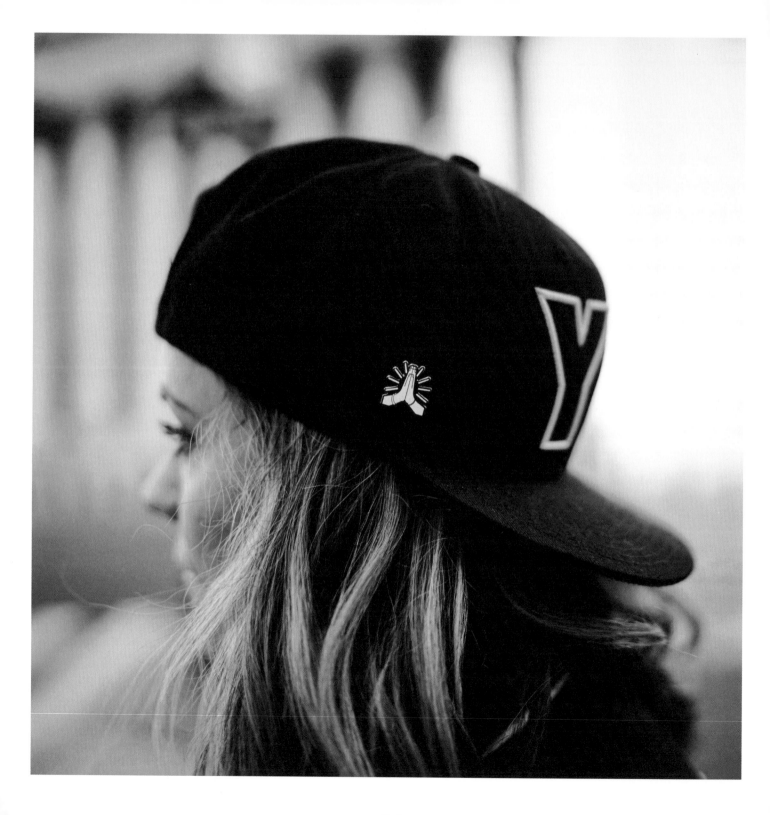

Index

A

Abs & Ass Sequence, 112–127
    Balancing Tabletop, 116, 117
    Boat Pose, 123
    Chair Pose, 121, 122
    Child's Pose, 114
    Downward Dog Split, 119
    Downward Facing Dog, 118
    High Lunge, 120
    Low Boat Pose, 124
    Playlist, 53
    Tabletop, 115
    Twisted Chair, 122
Alignment, 25
Asana, 32, 33, 134
Ashtanga, 31, 35
Awareness, 25, 32, 135

B

Balance, finding, 6, 22, 130–148, 150–167
Balancing Tabletop, 116, 117, 196
Bikram, 22, 31, 35
Bio-individuality, 144–147
Blood flow, stimulating, 26
Boat Pose, 123, 196
Body, caring for, 150–167
Body, nourishing, 143–148
Body–mind connection, 32, 35, 131, 135, 170
Bone health, 26
Boundaries, setting, 141
Brathen, Rachel, 17
Breathing exercise, 141

Breathing patterns, 32, 50, 57, 134
Breathing techniques, 22, 25, 26, 179–180, 186

C

Candlelight, 7, 19, 35–36, 39, 137
Cat Pose, 62, 196
Centering techniques, 6, 42, 141
Chair Pose, 121, 122, 196
Chair Twist, 107, 196
Chaturanga Dandasana, 71, 80, 91, 196
Child's Pose, 60–61, 114, 196
Closed Prayer Twist High Lunge, 106, 196
Cow Pose, 61, 62, 197
Crow Pose, 109, 197

D

Detox, 26, 57, 97, 145–147. See also Y7 Mega Detox
Dharana, 32
Dhyana, 32
DiDonato, Emily, 7
Diet, 143–148. See also Recipes
Digestion, improving, 26
Dirgha breath, 179, 180
Discipline, 141
Distractions, 140–141
Divers Pose, 108, 197
Downward Dog Split, 64, 83, 98, 100, 102, 119, 197
Downward Facing Dog, 63, 73, 78, 82, 92, 118, 198

E

Energy, increasing, 6, 25, 144–148
Enlightenment, 22, 32

F

Fallen Triangle, 101, 198
Flexibility, increasing, 22, 25
Flow guidelines, 46–47
Flow workout types, 48–50. *See also specific workouts*
Forward Fold, 67, 69, 90, 198

G

Glossary, 196–199
Gratitude, 137, 179, 180

H

Half Moon Pose, 88, 198
Halfway Lift, 69, 90, 198
Harmony, 31–32, 35, 131
Hatha practice, 33
Health, improving, 22, 25, 26, 143–148, 150–167
High Lunge, 85, 103, 120, 198
High Lunge T-Twist, 104, 198
Hip-hop music, 36–43, 47. *See also* Music playlists
Hip-hop yoga, 31–32, 36–37. *See also* Yoga
Hydration, 148

I

Immune system, 26
Inner peace, 17, 138

K

Karma, 31
Kundalini, 31

L

Laspina, Stephanie, 96–97
Levey, Mason, 7, 11, 13–14, 36
Levey, Sarah, 7, 11, 13–14, 58–59, 167, 171
Lewis, Kristin, 112–113
Love, 137–138
Low Boat Pose, 124, 198
Low Lunge, 65, 84, 198

M

Mantras, 134
Martini, Michelle, 171
Meditation
    benefits of, 169–176
    daily meditation, 179–180
    history of, 172–175
    moments for, 180
    moving meditation, 35
    poses for, 175–176
    sacred space for, 175–176
    unplugging for, 140–141
    Yoga Nidra, 183–191
Mental health, 19, 22, 152–153, 171–179
Mind, nourishing, 168–191
Mind–body connection, 32, 35, 131, 135, 170
Motivation, 22, 37–41, 152
Mountain Pose, 68, 198
Music, 19, 36–53
Music guidelines, 47
Music playlists, 43–47, 49–53

N

Negative thoughts, 137, 152–153
Nichols, Kristen, 76–77
Niyamas, 32
Nutrition, 143–148. *See also* Recipes

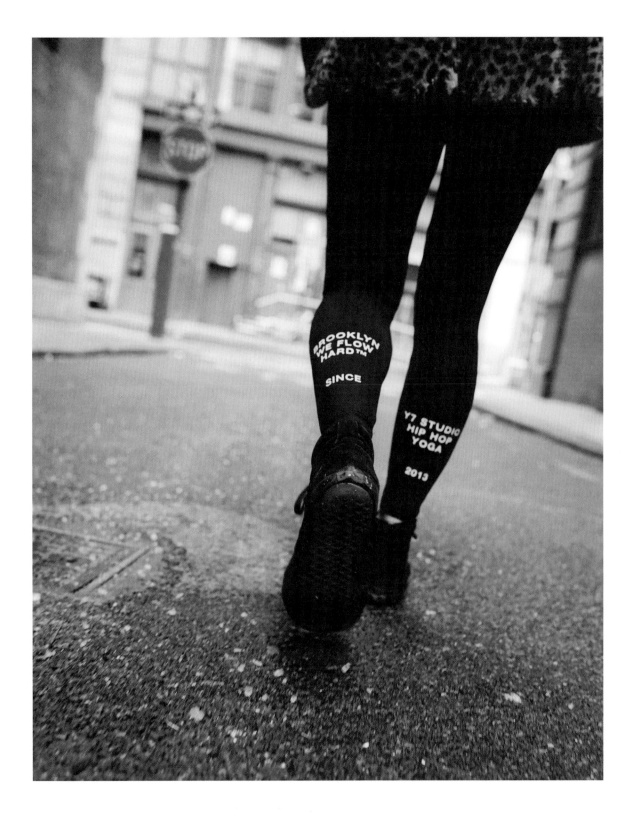

P

Pascal, Blaise, 171
Peace, 17, 138
Philosophy, 16–19, 131–133
Plank Pose, 70, 79, 92, 199
Playlists, 43–47, 49–53
Poses. *See also specific poses*
    for Abs & Ass Sequence, 112–127
    explanation of, 54–57
    glossary of, 196–199
    guidelines for, 46–47
    for Warm-up Sequence, 58–75
    for Y7 Flow, 76–95
    for Y7 Mega Detox, 96–111
Positive thoughts, 137, 152–153
Posture, 25, 32
Posture guidelines, 46–47
Pranayama, 32, 57, 134
Pratyahara, 32
Present moment, 25, 35, 42, 135, 141
Pyramid Pose, 66, 199

R

Recipes, 154–167
    Beverages, 165–167
    Breakfast Bowl, 156
    Breakfast Recipes, 155–156
    Caprese Salad on Crack, 159
    Cauliflower Breadsticks, 164
    Chicken with Beer, Honey, and Lime, 162
    Cocktails, 165–167
    Dinner Recipes, 160–162
    Lunch Recipes, 157–159
    Mescal Chill, 165
    Oats with Berries, 155
    Salmon with Garlic Butter, 160–161
    Sarah's Go-To Drink, 167
    Snacks, 163–164
    Tuna Salad Lettuce Wraps, 157
Restorative Flow playlist, 50
Restorative Flow workout, 50

Reverse Warrior, 86, 199
Revolved Peaceful Warrior, 105, 199
Rockstar Pose, 99, 199

S

Samadhi, 32
Sankalpa, 183, 184, 191
Self-care, 150–167
Self-confidence, 137–138
Self-discovery, 144–147
Self-doubt, 137
Self-love, 137–138, 176
Shankar, Ravi, 169
Staff Pose, 71
Strength training, 22
Stress, 140–141, 171–172
Stress relief, 22, 26, 169–175, 179–180
Support system, 152
Sutras, 134

T

Tabletop, 61, 115, 199
Triangle Pose, 87, 199
Twisted Chair, 122, 199

U

Unplugging, 25, 57, 140–141
Upward Facing Dog, 72, 81, 92, 199

V

Vinyasa, 22, 25, 31, 33, 35, 49–50
Vinyasa Flow, 25, 49, 55–57, 92
Vinyasa Flow playlist, 49
Vinyasa Flow workout, 49

W

Warm-up Sequence, 58–75
    Cat Pose, 62
    Chaturanga Dandasana, 71
    Child's Pose, 60–61

Cow Pose, 61, 62
Downward Dog Split, 64
Downward Facing Dog, 63, 73
Forward Fold, 67, 69
Halfway Lift, 69
Low Lunge, 65
Mountain Pose, 68
Plank Pose, 70
Playlist, 53
Pyramid Pose, 66
Staff Pose, 71
Tabletop, 61
Upward Facing Dog, 72
Warrior Two, 86, 89, 199
Water, drinking, 148
Weight loss, 22
Well-being, 21, 152–153
Workout types, 48–50. *See also specific*
workouts

Y

Y7 Flow, 76–95
Chaturanga Dandasana, 80, 91
Downward Dog Split, 83
Downward Facing Dog, 78, 82, 92
Forward Fold, 90
Half Moon Pose, 88
Halfway Lift, 90
High Lunge, 85
Low Lunge, 84
Plank Pose, 79, 92
Playlist, 53
Reverse Warrior, 86
Triangle Pose, 87
Upward Facing Dog, 81, 92
Vinyasa Flow, 92
Warrior Two, 86, 89
Y7 Mega Detox, 96–111
Chair Twist, 107
Closed Prayer Twist High Lunge, 106
Crow Pose, 109
Divers Pose, 108

Downward Dog Split, 98, 100, 102
Fallen Triangle, 101
High Lunge, 103
High Lunge T-Twist, 104
Playlist, 53
Revolved Peaceful Warrior, 105
Rockstar Pose, 99
Y7 Studio
beginning of, 10–15
design of, 19
expansion of, 15
experience with, 6–7, 19, 21, 59
philosophy of, 16–19, 131–133
Yamas, 32
Yoga. *See also specific poses*
Abs & Ass Sequence, 112–127
benefits of, 20–26, 32
days off, 152
guidelines for, 46–47
hip-hop yoga, 31–32, 36–37
history of, 31
limbs of, 32
for meditation, 175–176
philosophy of, 16–19, 131–133
practicing, 11–15, 18–26, 39–41, 133–135
reasons for, 20–26
Warm-up Sequence, 58–75
Y7 Flow, 76–95
Y7 Mega Detox, 96–111
Yoga Nidra, 183–191

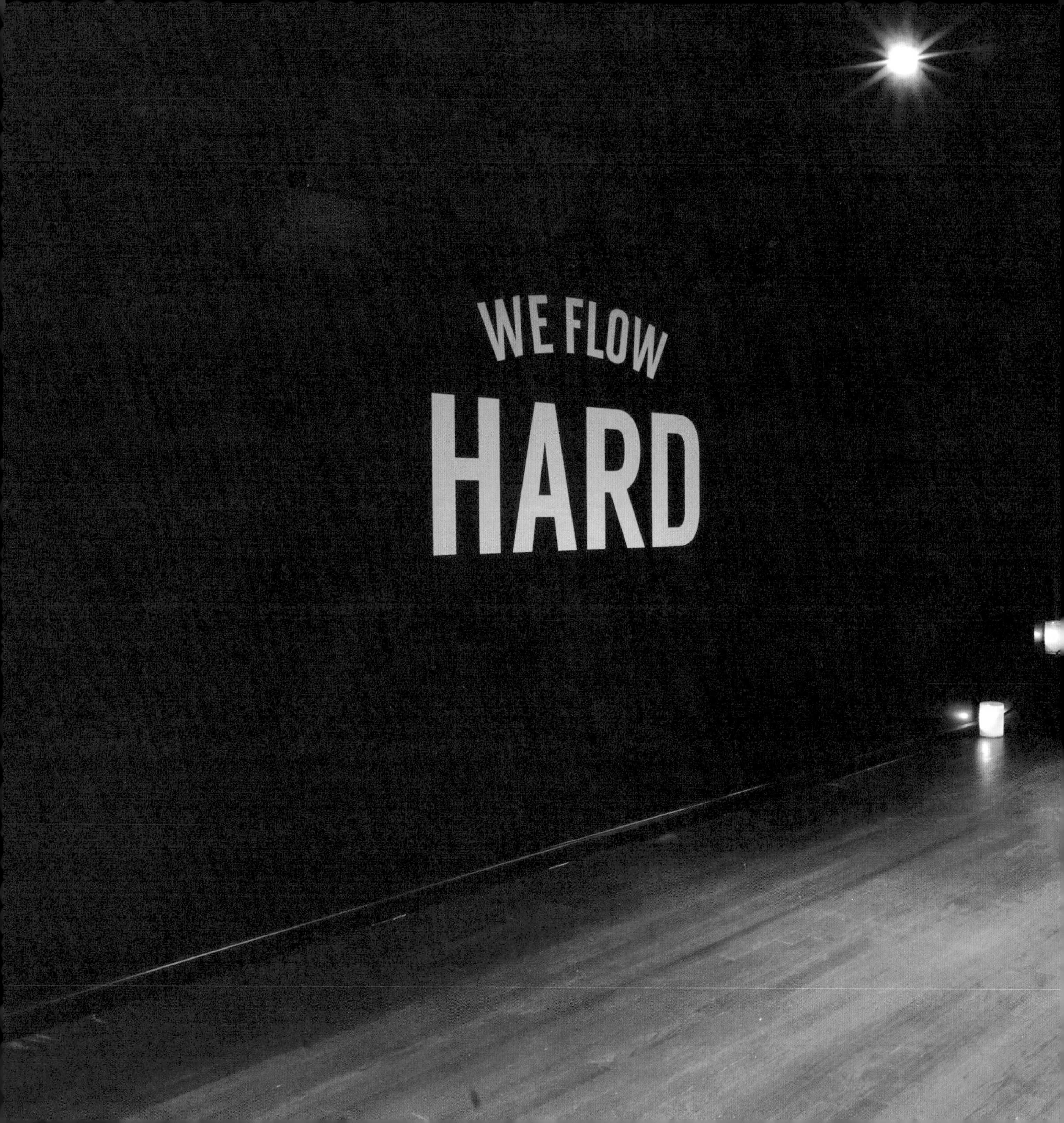
WE FLOW
HARD